EARLY-ONSET ALZHEIMER'S DISEASE
The Best Science in Everyday Language!

JERRY BELLER HEALTH RESEARCH INSTITUTE

Copyright © 2019 Jerry Beller
All rights reserved.
ISBN-13: 9781656820563

My diagnosis are Frontal Temperal Demencia and Posterior Cortical Atrophy

DEDICATION

To people living with Dementia and their loved ones.

CONTENTS

FOREWORD 1

Who is the reading audience? 5

I. DEMENTIA 16

Chapter 1: WHAT IS DEMENTIA? 17

Chapter 2: WHAT ARE THE 19 PRIMARY DEMENTIAS? 21

Chapter 3: WHO IS MOST LIKELY TO GET DEMENTIA? 23

Chapter 4: DEMENTIA COSTS & PREVALENCE 33

Chapter 5: 19 PRIMARY DEMENTIA TYPES 46

II. EARLY-ONSET ALZHEIMER'S DISEASE (EOAD) DEMENTIAS .49

Chapter 6: WHAT IS ALZHEIMER'S DISEASE? 50

III. EOAD SYMPTOMS 85

Chapter 8: EARLY-ONSET ALZHEIMER'S DISEASE (EOAD) SYMPTOMS 86

Chapter 9: EOAD SYMPTOMS 87

Chapter 10: EOAD STAGES 110

V. EOAD RELATED RISK FACTORS 130

Chapter 11: EOAD RISK FACTORS 131

VI. BONUS SECTION 194

Chapter 12: Starter To-do List for Somebody and Family once Diagnosed with Dementia. 195

Chapter 13: CARE TEAM 203

Chapter 14: LETTER TO CONGRESS 206

CONCLUSION 208

THANK YOU FOR READING 212

BELLER HEALTH BOOKS 213

Other Beller Health Books 216

ABOUT THE AUTHOR 217

ACKNOWLEDGMENTS

Thanks to the American Academy of Neurology, Atlanta Center for Medical Research, Alzheimer's Association, Alzheimer's Disease Center, Alzheimer's Disease Center of Northwestern University, Alzheimer's Foundation of America, American Academy of Neurology, Association for Frontotemporal Degeneration, Australia Neurological Research, CDC, Department of Health and Human Services, Duke University Medical Center, Emory Hospital, Harvard Medical School, Johns Hopkins Medicine, Mayo Clinic, National Aphasia Association, National Institute of Neurological Disorders and Strokes, National Library of Medicine, National Institute on Aging, National Institutes of Health, Prince of Wales Medical Research Institute, *PubMed*, Stanford Library School of Medicine, Stanford Medicine, UCSF Department of Neurology, UCSF Memory and Aging Center, University of Cambridge Neurology Unit, World Health Organization (WHO), *Journal of American Medical Association* (JAMA), and several other organizations that provided information used for this book. Thanks to everybody who assisted this book in a variety of important ways, and everybody at Beller Health Research Institute. To my editor, John Briggs, who helps me improve every book. To all sources and for the photos. Most of all, thanks to my wife, Nicola Beller

FOREWORD

Before diving into the book's subject matter, let's discuss two related Dementia series:

- *2020 Dementia Overview* series
- *2020 Dementia Types, Symptoms, Stages, & Risk Factors* series

2020 Dementia Overview series is an extension of the medical groundbreaking *19 Dementia Types, Symptoms, Stages, & Risk Factors* series, the first covering <u>all primary dementia types.</u>

After spending decades building an audience in other genres, including nutrition, circumstances turned the world upside down. Doctors diagnosed my mother with Alzheimer's. The same doctors soon diagnosed my father with cancer. A few months later, my father's favorite brother and my closest uncle died.

Three consecutive hard blows blew the world beyond recognition.

Tough and decent as they come, dad insisted on taking care of my mother while fighting brain cancer. My brothers and sister-in-law did their share, but Dad cared for my mother for a long time while they worked. Dad proved what a remarkable and great man he was down the stretch but finally succumbed to brain cancer.

My brothers and sister-in-law did their best to take care of mom, but it came at a price. Caregiving for a dementia patient is an indescribable horror I would not wish on my worst enemy.

You must watch somebody you love wilt away, little by little until dementia wipes away huge chunks of their personality.

Living away, my wife and I visited when possible. We saw how mom deteriorated, but also the effect caregiving had on my father and brothers. It was like watching a train wreck over and over, each time getting worse and helpless to prevent it.

Watching Alzheimer's takedown, my strong-willed mother and others bruised my soul. My writing shifted initially to learn about Alzheimer's, but the more learned, the more I cringed.

The cold hard facts rendered me speechless. Over 5.8 million Americans, and 44 million people worldwide, suffer Alzheimer's. No cure. Just a devastating and expensive slow march towards an agonizing end.

Not content to kill, Alzheimer's tortured Mom for years before killing her. It robbed her memory and damaged her brain, where she repeated herself in a continuous loop, each time thinking she was saying it the first time. As the disease advanced, the neurological disorder destroyed her mind and body.

Seeing dementia take down that tough old bird rattled me. While I could not bring back my mother, I dedicate my life to researching and writing about dementia 8-12 hours per day, six or seven days per week.

I tackled Alzheimer's to learn everything I could about the brute and determine how I and others might prevent it and other noncommunicable diseases. Having written on nutrition and advocated health in Washington, I already had a clue but determined to figure out how to prevent Alzheimer's. But I needed to know more, much more, about this terrorizing neurological disorder.

I learned Alzheimer's was just one of over one-hundred neurological disorders causing dementia. When I searched for a book covering the primary dementias, none existed. Instead, I turned to individual books and again found no books written on several of the most frequent dementias.

In what on the one hand seems like yesterday and the other a lifetime ago, I set out several years ago to write a dementia book covering the 15 most prevalent dementia types. The first to do that, I next wrote books covering each of the 15 most prevalent dementias.

In 2020, I expanded the book covering 15 dementias to 19 dementia types. I also released books on each of the 19 dementias. While proud of these medical firsts, I do not take myself too seriously.

As one of the dozens of scientists, neurologists, researchers, and writers who devote their lives to fighting the war against dementia, I remain humble. I appreciate the individual and combined accomplishments of everybody else in the field.

Nor should any of us get cocky knowing we're losing the war. If we win the war during my lifetime, I will celebrate with hundreds of people worldwide who helped defeat the great beast of our day.

My two-book series break medical ground, and I consider major achievements but remain two among hundreds of significant contributions to the dementia field by people around the globe.

The series provides patients and loved ones a great resource for dementias not covered as extensive as Alzheimer's and the more prevalent types.

By covering the 19 most prevalent dementias, doctors, nurses, and medical professionals benefit from a series covering neurological disorders causing 99% of dementia. The series helps primary care physicians, providers, and nurses who struggle to diagnose dementias with overlapping symptoms.

The series is an organic, evolving work, and each book receives major annual updates. As science uncovers information, we add important data in new editions. We also polish each edition.

We describe the writing goal in three ways:
1. Simplify the language and make it easier for nonscientists to comprehend.
2. Honor the science and facts.
3. Document science and include citations for doctors,

nurses, medical researchers, students, and patients.

Our goal is to provide invaluable medical information for professionals, patients, loved ones, and caregivers.

I do not reinvent the wheel but accumulate the best research and teach our readers a better understanding of Alzheimer's and the other 18 primary dementia types.

Among the worst news is one of our loved ones has dementia. A killer disease with no cure frightens the bravest souls.

This medical condition destroys, not just the inflicted, but their loved ones. Besides the patient, nobody suffers more than voluntary caregivers. Watching a mother, father, brother, sister, wife, or husband suffering dementia brutalizes the soul.

I study dementia year around to write and release annual updates to honor people—including my mother—taken by Alzheimer's or one of the other primary dementias.

Modest book royalties are the only compensation, as I accept no money from corporations to promote their product. Nor do I have an ax to grind with anybody in the medical profession.

Having written 100 plus books over four decades, I am thankful to readers for collectively providing me a decent income. However, now in my sixties, I care little about riches and fame.

Who is the reading audience?

The audience falls into five categories.

Those Diagnosed with Dementia

If doctors diagnose you with dementia, my heart goes out to you. You're in for a long battle. Do yourself a favor and focus on slowing the disease and extending the quality of life. One word of caution, the books in this series speak to not only patients, but also families, doctors, students, nurses, and caregivers. Many of those diagnosed with dementia appreciate and benefit from the books, but some find some of the material too disturbing. I intend to write books exclusively for patients but must finish the work related to this series first. While there is not anything too shocking, I wrote the material for a wide audience, meaning I am not always speaking to patients specifically. I promise to personalize an edition for patients and loved ones after finishing this series. By shining a light on all 19 primary dementia types, I hope to help the medical community better distinguish and diagnose neurological disorders.

Loved Ones of Those Diagnosed

If doctors diagnose a loved one with dementia, he or she needs you more than ever. Depending on the type, dementia causes behavioral problems, memory issues, motor decline, and other psychological and physical disorders. The learning curve is steep and changes as one moves from one stage to the next. As with those with dementia, I warn families these books provide a technical overview, and the emphasis is not always on the emotional aspect. If you want to learn about dementias, this series is a great option. If you're looking more for emotional support, there are more appropriate books. I also plan to write a book specifically for families once fulfilling responsibilities for this series.

Medical Professionals

If you are a medical professional interested in studying the dementias, the series covers the dementias responsible for 99% of dementia. While neurologists probably already know the 19 primary dementias, the books provide a quick overview and reference for primary care physicians, nurses, other medical professionals, and students. I also include citations so you can continue your investigation beyond the book's scope.

Volunteer & Professional Caregivers

If you are a dementia caregiver, you are also in for a long, difficult march. Dementia patients demand 24/7 care in later stages, requiring help to go to the bathroom, bathing, and other basic daily functions. While this series is not written solely for caregiving, caregivers benefit by gaining a better understanding of each dementia, their symptoms, and progression.

Anybody Wanting to Learn About A Disease That Strikes 1 Of 6 Americans, And 1 Of 3 Seniors

The series benefits anybody who wants to gain an intermediate understanding of the 19 dementias.

Series' First Lesson

Doctors, like teachers, are part of a sacred profession. **Nothing I say or write replaces your need for a competent doctor!** Nor does any criticism of the profession diminish my respect and admiration for the best.

I detest the worst teachers who fail students and society but love and respect the best. Society would crumble without the most devoted and competent teachers.

Similar, I abhor incompetent, greedy doctors who fail patients and society, but love and respect the best.

The profession must weed out incompetent, uncaring, corrupt doctors, and medical personnel. Every profession has a percentage of bad apples, but within the medical profession, they are cancerous!

Nothing good I write about the medical profession includes incompetent, uncaring doctors, researchers, nurses, etc. And nothing bad I write targets the best.

The series criticizes the profession when deserved, but the first lesson in this series: **Find a competent doctor!** If you have one, count your blessings. If not, find one.

Just as one can learn outside the classroom, we live in a blessed age where medical information is available for anybody on the internet. Such information serves us well, but do not—for a minute-think it replaces the need for a competent, devoted doctor.

The Wrong Doctors

Let me begin this section by saying I love and respect quality doctors, nurses, researchers, and medical professionals from the bottom of my heart and the fullness of my mind.

However, this section is not about what's right in the medical profession.

Glorified idiots, bad doctors are dangerous parasites who dishonor a noble profession. Smart enough to finish medical school, but greedy or flawed beyond redemption, they are like priests working for the devil. Among the worse members of society are doctors motivated by greed or limited by incompetence. Walking parasites!

The Wrong Doctors + Big Pharm + Big Insurance + Big Hospital = Expensive & Inadequate Health Care

Over the past few decades, Big pharmaceuticals, Big Insurance, and their political puppets appointed doctors sanctioned drug dealers. Entrusting the worse doctors with such powers produces little or no better results than assigning the task to a thug on the worst corner in America.

The worst doctors who hand out drugs like candy serve nobody's purpose but their own and Big Pharm.

Not an indictment of the entire profession, but unfortunately, Big Insurance dictates the typical office visit includes a quick examination and one or more prescriptions. The approach is not based on good science and runs counter to everything science teaches us.

What About Some Tough Love?

The one thing people today do not want is what we often need most, tough love. People want everything sugarcoated and easy.

The problem is most of the time; life is neither sweet nor easy.

What patients need much of the time is not an alleged "magic pill," but instead tough love. Doctors must learn nutrition and teach patients to eat healthier, exercise more, and get 7-8 hours of sleep per night. Like it or not, this is part of modern medicine. Showing up and passing out pills all day is not preventing Alzheimer's and other dementias, nor curing them.

Medical professionals must lead by example and embrace the science of nutrition, exercise, and sleep. If a healthy diet and exercise are the two cornerstones to health, the third is sleep.

The average person needs few or no drugs if they practice healthy habits.

Any doctor who does not vigorously advocate a balanced whole food diet, exercise most days of the week, and 7-8 hours' sleep per night neglects their duty and

Instead, too many doctors ignore the three cornerstones of health and are content to write their patients unnecessary and potentially dangerous prescriptions for the rest of their lives. 100% emphasis on treating symptoms with drugs, which often require more drugs to counter the side effects, is producing disastrous results. To be the best doctor, one must also emphasize prevention.

Failed Drug Trials

None of the drug trials have produced even one drug that cures Alzheimer's and other dementias. While science has failed to produce any effective dementia drugs, scientific studies prove we can do much by practicing healthy habits to slow or reduce our dementia risk.

The Medical Profession Must Think Outside The Box

The hopeless circle of failed drug trials demands we think outside the box or, as neurologist David Perlmutter advocates, expand the box. He and other neurologists deserve credit for recognizing medicine is failing the dementia war and rocking the boat of conventional wisdom. I must not agree with every point "maverick" neurologists like David Perlmutter, Dale Bredesen, and Deepak Chopra make to respect them for turning conventional wisdom on its head.

Conventional wisdom is losing the Alzheimer's and dementia war!

Not Anti-doctors or Anti-drugs

I am not anti-doctors or anti-drugs and do not understand those who insist neither are needed. I revere competent doctors who practice and advocate the three cornerstones of health. I also recognize the polio vaccine and many other drugs as nothing short of miraculous.

But, my love for what is right about the medical profession will not silence me about what is wrong. And, pretending drugs are the answer to defeating Alzheimer's or dementia is a colossal failure.

You cannot "**do no harm**" and write prescription drugs at the volume of the average doctor.

Choose A Doctor with The Same Care As You Do A Spouse

Find a competent, dedicated, caring, experienced, informed, ethical doctor who listens and respects your opinion, and writes prescriptions as a LAST RESORT.

Without the right doctor, you are at the mercy of a profit-oriented health system that seldom puts the patient's interests first, second, or third.

Nothing I say or write in these books or elsewhere means you should not see a doctor, stop taking your medication, or otherwise undermine the medical profession's ability to diagnose and treat any medical symptoms you might experience.

Find a good doctor you trust with your life and ask him or her pointed questions concerning your health and any treatment they recommend.

Outside the Bubble

I challenge the medical profession where necessary, just as I criticize Congress and the United States government for their mistakes or shortcomings. My brief career as a Congressional staffer taught me how difficult it is to maintain one's focus inside the bubble.

Seeing the big picture is no less challenging inside the medical bubble motivated by profit.

Profiteers fund too many studies to promote their product or discredit somebody else's. Blatant self-interests taint studies and confuse the public. Such contradictory studies confuse and make it impossible for the average person to understand which studies to believe.

I respect ethical, competent, dedicated, and hardworking nurses, doctors, and other medical personnel. As much as I criticize what is wrong within the profession, I cannot praise the majority of medical professionals often enough. Getting quality medical care when we need it is one of life's greatest blessings.

Nor do I object to medical-related businesses making a reasonable profit in return for needed medical supplies and services.

Nor should any competent and ethical medical professionals object to anybody challenging medical incompetence and profiteers.

Trust Thy Doctor

The right doctor does not discriminate between physical and mental diseases, so hold back nothing if you or a loved one exhibits symptoms.

If you lack the right doctor, find the right one. Outside you and the daily habits you establish, nobody is more important than your doctor for your health. You must be able to tell him or her medical information you might be reluctant to tell your closest confidant in life.

Remember, doctors too often misdiagnose dementia. Once the symptoms of these deadly dementias set in, you need to see your doctor, provide them with all the information about your problem, and help the specialists reach the correct diagnosis.

Because no tests exist for most dementias, doctors order tests and go through a process of elimination until reaching a diagnosis based on the symptoms you report. The more information you provide, the better the chance of a quick and accurate diagnosis.

Adopt healthy lifestyle choices to prevent dementia when possible, but the next best option is to diagnose it early, to confront it head-on, and take steps to slow the disease. Once dementia hits, it's often possible to postpone the advanced stages. If you've seen a loved one inflicted with dementia, you understand how precious a year, a month, a week, or day is once the storm aims at you or a loved one.

Prolonging life in late-stage dementia without a cure amounts to cruel and unusual punishment, but patients, families, and doctors must do everything possible to extend quality of life while possible.

Make certain you have a doctor who believes in prevention and natural cures, but also remember you need their expertise concerning the best that modern medicine offers.

Be Your Nurse!

If you have a loved one, be each other's nurse. If not, be your nurse.

It's more important than ever for you to monitor your blood pressure and make notes of health issues as they arise. We don't go to the doctor every time we develop a symptom or don't feel well, but it's important to keep a medical journal. Write an outline of the problems you experience between visits.

Too often, we march into the physician's office and don't provide a full or accurate representation of our problem. For instance, if you track your blood pressure, you can furnish a pattern rather than a onetime reading. You can also perhaps attribute pikes in your blood pressure to stress taking place in your life.

You should also track other symptoms. Providing thorough information helps doctors eliminate multiple diseases with similar symptoms. When you document all or most of the symptoms that have led to the visit, you provide a competent doctor a clearer picture to develop a hypothesis. These previous unrelated symptoms might help your physician make more sense of what prompted the appointment.

Otherwise, your physician might order the wrong tests or prescribe the wrong drugs. For issues of the brain, you can't be shy or embarrassed about providing your physician with a full portrayal of your problems and symptoms.

Although still stigmatized in some circles, mental illnesses are just as real, and the sufferers are no more the blame, than physical disorders. While we must do everything in our power to avoid or slow mental or physical maladies, the last thing we need to do is embarrass those who are already suffering.

Two Dementia Series

The laborious task to document the primary dementias began as a fifty-page Alzheimer's overview. Two editions later, the 50-page Alzheimer's book turned into 400 pages.

One of the first lessons taught Alzheimer's is only one of the hundreds of diseases responsible for dementia. With inadequate testing, similar symptoms, and other handicaps, the medical community often misdiagnoses the other dementias for Alzheimer's.

My focus broadened from Alzheimer's to a dozen dementias. The only way to make any sense of Alzheimer's or dementia was to study all the primary dementias.

I worked with several neurologists and researchers over the next couple of years and hit every medical library I could hit in person or available online.

After an extensive review, I wrote the first book covering the 15 most prevalent dementia types, which provided the groundwork for two updated dementia series.

The associated *Dementia Types, Symptoms, Stages, & Risk Factors, series* expands the collection by adding amyotrophic lateral sclerosis (ALS), early-onset Alzheimer's disease, amyotrophic lateral sclerosis, corticobasal syndrome, and progressive supranuclear palsy.

Two Dementia Series

Not counting mixed dementia, there are nineteen primary dementia types, which two groundbreaking series covers.

Dementia Types, Symptoms, Stages, & Risk Factors series

1. Dementia with Lewy Bodies
2. Parkinson's Disease Dementia
3. Corticobasal Syndrome
4. Typical Alzheimer's Disease
5. Posterior Cortical Atrophy
6. Down Syndrome with Alzheimer's
7. Limbic-predominant Age-related TDP-43 Encephalopathy (LATE)
8. Early-onset Alzheimer's
9. Behavioral Variant Frontotemporal Dementia
10. Progressive Supranuclear Palsy
11. Nonfluent Primary Progressive Aphasia
12. Logopenic Progressive Aphasia
13. Cortical Vascular Dementia
14. Binswanger Disease
15. Normal Pressure Hydrocephalus
16. Huntington's Disease
17. Korsakoff Syndrome
18. Creutzfeldt-Jakob Disease
19. Amyotrophic Lateral Sclerosis

*Not a dementia type, but a combination, mixed dementia is the 20th category important in dementia discussions.

Any disease leading to associated symptoms is a dementia type. The series breaks medical ground by covering the dementias responsible for over 99% of dementia cases.

EARLY-ONSET ALZHEIMER'S DISEASE (EOAD)

2020 Dementia Overview Series

The second series focuses on all the primary dementia types or breaks them down as groups.

1. <u>Dementia Types, Symptoms, & Stages</u>
2. <u>Lewy Body/Parkinsonism Dementias</u>
3. <u>Vascular Dementia</u>
4. <u>Frontotemporal Dementia (FTD)</u>
5. <u>Alzheimer's Related Dementias</u>
6. <u>Prevent or Slow Dementia</u>

I. DEMENTIA

In this section, we discuss dementia.

Dementia is not a disease but a medical condition. Hundreds of diseases and disorders lead to dementia, but percentage-wise, almost all dementia falls under 19 primary dementia categories.

This series is the first to cover all 19 primary dementia types.

In this chapter, we answer the following questions:
- What is dementia?
- What are the 19 primary dementias?
- How prevalent is dementia?
- Who is most likely to get dementia?
- What are the financial costs to individuals, the U.S., and worldwide?

Once we answer these questions and provide a dementia overview, we turn our attention to the subject matter for the rest of the book.

Let's begin by answering the question: What is dementia?

Chapter 1: WHAT IS DEMENTIA?

For centuries, when one got dementia, people described the person in terms like "gone mad," or "lost their mind," or "crazy," or another derogatory term that missed the mark.

While most dementia types attack cognitive skills and cause behavioral disorders, the person is no less a victim than a cancer patient.

Whereas cancer attacks cells and organs, dementia destroys brain neurons.

The brain is complex. One-hundred billion neurons use over 100 trillion synapses and about 100 neurotransmitters to send all the signals to other parts of the brain, organs, and parts throughout the body, allowing us to think, reason, walk, talk, breathe, and do all that makes us human.

When fed, protected, and healthy, neurons perform magic.

The different dementias attack the brain and destroy the communication network responsible for everything our body does. By attacking different parts of the brain, the dementia types cause different disorders.

Let's see how some of the most prestigious American and global medical organizations define Dementia.

Alzheimer's Association Definition

Let's begin with the Alzheimer's Association:

> *Dementia is an overall term for diseases and conditions characterized by a decline in memory, language, problem-solving, and other thinking skills that affect a person's ability to perform everyday activities. Memory loss is an example. Alzheimer's is the most common cause of dementia*[1].

Dementia is to Alzheimer's, dementia with Lewy bodies,

Parkinson's dementia, vascular and the other dementia types what Asia is to China, India, North Korea, South Korea, and the rest of Asia. Alzheimer's is the most prevalent dementia, but each type devastates, and most are death sentences.

Let's turn to the National Institute on Aging (NIH) and see how they define dementia.

National Institute on Aging (NIH)

The National Institute on Aging (NIH) funds many studies and provides researchers invaluable data. How do they define dementia?

> *Dementia is the loss of cognitive functioning – thinking, remembering, and reasoning – and behavioral abilities to such an extent that it interferes with a person's daily life and activities. These functions include memory, language skills, visual perception, problem-solving, self-management, and the ability to focus and pay attention. Some people with dementia cannot control their emotions, and their personalities may change. Dementia ranges in severity from the mildest stage, when it is just beginning to affect a person's functioning, to the most severe stage, when the person must depend completely on others for basic activities of living*[2].

One of the most important things a person and their loved ones can do when diagnosed with dementia; enjoy what quality time remains.

Early diagnosis, medication, and lifestyle changes can slow the disease and extend quality life. From the point of diagnosis, make the most of each good day or moment.

Let's see how the international community defines dementia.

Alzheimer's Society UK

The Alzheimer's Society is perhaps the UK's most

prestigious Alzheimer's organization. They define dementia:

> *The word 'dementia' describes a set of symptoms that may include memory loss and difficulties with thinking, problem-solving or language. These changes are often small to start with, but for someone with dementia they have become severe enough to affect daily life. A person with dementia may also experience changes in their mood or behaviour[3].*

Let's see how the World Health Organization (WHO) defines dementia.

World Health Organization (WHO)

The World Health Organization (WHO) works with global medical organizations and provides researchers a wealth of information. How does WHO define dementia?

> *Dementia is a syndrome – usually of a chronic or progressive nature – in which there is deterioration in cognitive function (i.e. the ability to process thought) beyond what might be expected from normal ageing. It affects memory, thinking, orientation, comprehension, calculation, learning capacity, language, and judgement. Consciousness is not affected. The impairment in cognitive function is commonly accompanied, and occasionally preceded, by deterioration in emotional control, social behaviour, or motivation[4].*

The four organizations provide similar definitions, each emphasizing different points, but none contradicting the others.

Each organization confirms dementia is a broad neurological disorder. Hundreds of pathologies such as Alzheimer's leads to dementia, but 19 primary types cause about 99% of dementia cases. Dementia attacks the brain and causes memory decline, behavior disorders, motor decline, language deterioration, and most types are incurable.

If doctors diagnose you with dementia, you must get past the shock. Time is moving against you, so make the most of it.

As the Alzheimer's Society points out, the symptoms are minor in the beginning. Get your affairs in order, enjoy loved ones, and take part in as many activities as you desire and are able. To some extent, this is your farewell tour. Take advantage!

The disease will stop you or a loved one later, so do not stop living your life in the early stages.

Let's next examine the 19 primary dementia types.

Chapter 2: WHAT ARE THE 19 PRIMARY DEMENTIAS?

Hundreds of medical conditions lead to dementia, but 19 causes up to 99% of cases.

Each dementia type is devastating, most are fatal, and the first symptoms to death is a challenging, heartbreaking, soul-crushing experience. Dementia robs the personalities and functionality of marvelous people a little at a time until they no longer resemble the person they've always been.

19 Dementia Types

This chapter divides the 19 primary dementias into six categories. The first group includes dementias related to Lewy body or Parkinsonism dementia. The second consists of Alzheimer's-related dementia. In the third, we focus on primary progressive aphasia dementias. The fourth contains vascular dementias. The fifth category encompasses the remaining dementias and is called *other dementias*.

Lewy Body/Parkinsonism Related Dementias

1. *Dementia with Lewy Bodies*
2. *Parkinson's Disease Dementia*
3. Corticobasal Syndrome

Alzheimer's Related Dementias

4. Typical Alzheimer's Disease
5. Posterior Cortical Atrophy
6. Down Syndrome with Alzheimer's
7. Limbic-predominant Age-related TDP-43 Encephalopathy (LATE)
8. Early-onset Alzheimer's

Frontotemporal Lobar Degeneration Related Dementias

9. *Behavioral Variant Frontotemporal Dementia*
10. Progressive Supranuclear Palsy

Primary Progressive Aphasia Related Dementias

11. *Nonfluent Primary Progressive Aphasia (nfvPPA)*
12. Logopenic Progressive Aphasia (LPA)

Vascular Dementia

13. *Cortical Vascular Dementia*
14. *Binswanger Disease*

Other Dementias

15. *Normal Pressure Hydrocephalus*
16. *Huntington's Disease*
17. *Korsakoff Syndrome*
18. *Creutzfeldt-Jakob Disease*
19. Amyotrophic Lateral Sclerosis

Chapter 3: WHO IS MOST LIKELY TO GET DEMENTIA?

In this chapter, we explore who is most likely to get dementia. Most know people with dementia are old, but some people are born with dementia, others get it as infants, and the disease attacks people in every age group.

There are risk factors that affect everybody. Examples include a poor diet, lack of exercise, diabetes, obesity, high blood pressure, and factors under and beyond our control.

In this chapter, we focus on risk factors affecting specific groups of people who suffer higher rates.

The research pointed to age, race, and sex, where dementia seems to discriminate. Let's review the science for each.

Age

Age is the obvious risk factor. We know because of science and our observations.

So associated with the elderly, many believe dementia only strikes older people. However, dementia strikes all ages and demographics, including newborns and infants.

According to Stanford University Medical School, "The risk of Alzheimer's disease, vascular dementia, and several other dementias goes up significantly with advancing age[5]."

None of us enjoy aging. We must work harder and harder to slow aging, and no matter how well we do, none of us will make it much past 100 years. The better we take care of ourselves, the higher chance we have of living a quality life into our eighties or nineties.

Remember, aging does not destroy our cognitive abilities. Bad habits do! I stress this point because each of us can slow the aging process through healthy habits.

As people age, however, our dementia risks increase.

A Journal of Neurology, Neurosurgery, & Psychiatry study

concluded[6]:

> In the age group 65–69 years, there are more than two new cases per 1000 persons every year. This number increases almost exponentially with increasing age, until over the age of 90 years, out of 1000 persons, 70 new cases of dementia can be expected every year.

As we stress in our book on prevention, there is actual age and real age. We determine one's actual age by the day and year born, whereas weight, blood pressure, blood sugar, cholesterol, diet, how often you work out, and several other important factors govern our real age.

Unless genes or an accident prevents us, our real age should be lower than our actual age. Those who practice bad habits, however, raise their real age ten years or more than their actual age.

When our real age is lower than our actual age, we lower our risks for dementia and other diseases. When our real age is higher than our actual age, we increase risks for dementia, heart disease, cancer, and all major diseases.

Let's next review if race plays a role in dementia.

Race

African Americans and blacks in western countries suffer more than their share of racism.

The United States has abused too many citizens since its creation, but none more than Native Americans and African Americans.

But, does dementia also discriminate against them?

According to AARP, African Americans are 64% more likely to get dementia than non-Hispanic whites[7].

Kaiser Permanente Study

Researchers in another study examined data from 274,000

Kaiser Permanente patients over 14 years. They found the highest rate of dementia for African Americans and Native Americans[8].

Dementia Risk Per 1,000 People
- 27 African Americans
- 22 Native Americans
- 20 Latinos and Pacific Islanders
- 19 White Americans
- 15 Asian-Americans

Does dementia love Asian and European-Americans and hate African and Native-Americans?

Dementia is as evil as the worst bigot, but dementia is not a bigot.

African Americans experience higher rates of diabetes. African Americans and Native Americans suffer a higher level of stress, poverty, and disenfranchisement. Both cultures also struggle with their people's history in European-America and endure a greater level of bigotry and more obstacles to succeeding in modern America.

On the flip side, Asian Americans and whites have lower obesity and diabetes rates, eat a more balanced diet, faceless bigotry, are more affluent, educated, and successful in modern America.

We need more studies to confirm the exact causes of higher dementia incidence in the African and Native American populations. Higher stress and diabetes in their communities are prime suspects.

Jennifer Manly, Columbia University, Taub Institute for Research on Alzheimer's disease, and Aging Brain spoke to Reuters about the inequities.

There are huge disparities in dementia that are confronting this nation and this will translate into an enormous burden on families if we don't address this. We need to prioritize research that uncovers the reasons for these disparities and more research should include racially and ethnically diverse people[9].

Are African British at a greater risk for Dementia?

In the United Kingdom, black women are 25% more likely than white women, and black men 28% more likely than white men to get dementia[10].

Reluctance to Take Part in Dementia Studies

African Americans and Native Americans are also less trustful of studies. Too often in the past, a bigoted establishment treated African Americans and Native Americans like lab rats.

The awful past makes the average African American reluctant to take part in studies that might help us figure out how to lower the rates.

Native Americans are also distrustful of the United States government and the "white man's studies," as one group from the Cherokee Reservation in North Carolina told me.

I understand both ethnic groups' skepticism. As somebody with ancestors who died and survived the Trail of Tears, and who married a black woman (30+ years), nobody must convince me of the tainted American history. I have read about the past and viewed enough with my own eyes to know the sins of America's past, either haunt or still torment today.

But, the Studies are Necessary!

I call on African Americans and Native Americans to take part in dementia studies. The studies today have greater safeguards than the past and face much more scrutiny.

Dementia is a death sentence!

Worse than the average killer, never content to kill and move on, dementia is a sadist. Dementia destroys the mind and body, little by little, robbing one's personality, dignity, mind, body, and everything that makes a person unique.

If African Americans and Native Americans refuse to participate in dementia studies, fatal neurological disorders will continue to strike them worse than other ethnic groups.

Please consider two facts.

If you do not have dementia, researchers do not subject you to drug trials but accumulate data to determine which habits increase and decrease one's risks.

If doctors diagnose you with dementia, trials represent your last best chance to win what is otherwise a losing battle.

What Role does Poverty Play?

Although not listed as a dementia risk factor, poverty increases one's risk for almost every significant disease. Those at the bottom must worry where the next meal is coming, if somebody might mug (or kill) them when leaving the house, and a laundry list of stress the average citizen seems oblivious.

Beller Health calls for more research to determine if Native American, African American, and African British citizens have higher dementia rates as a general population, or if poverty drives these numbers. We need to know whether the number also applies to middle-and upper-class African Americans and Native Americans who eat healthily, exercise, do not abuse alcohol, avoid tobacco, and do not abuse prescription or illicit drugs.

Native American, African American, and African British citizens suffer a higher percentage of poverty than other demographics in the US and UK.

Rather than race, such factors as poverty, bigotry, and lack of opportunities might drive these numbers.

I reached out to several organizations, including the VA, to conduct a large-scale study to determine what role poverty plays in dementia. Most organizations greeted my request with enthusiasm, and I hope one or more soon back the study.

All we know for certain is poverty in the industrial world causes a much greater level of stress and other hardships than the rest of the population. WHO reported that about 60% of dementia cases occur in the poorest half of countries[11].

Age and ethnicity are dementia risk factors. What about sex?

Sex

Dementia strikes older people, African Americans, Native Americans, and African British in greater numbers than the rest of the population. Does one's gender increase or decrease one's odds?

How Many Women have Dementia?

According to the Alzheimer's Association, women represent two-thirds of people living with Alzheimer's, and 13 million women suffer dementia or are caring for somebody who does[12].

Of the 820,000 people living with dementia in the UK, females account for 61 percent[13].

Of the 50 million people living with dementia worldwide[14], women represent 65 percent[15].

Key points:

- Women represent two-thirds of Alzheimer's cases.
- Females account for 65% of dementia cases.

Is dementia just another woman-hating predator?

Does Alzheimer's & Most Dementia Strike Women in Greater Numbers?

While the two key numbers suggest dementia is a rampaging woman-abusing murderer, the answer is not so simple.

While women represent two-thirds of Alzheimer's cases and 65% of dementia cases, there are 19 primary dementia types.

Some dementias attack men in greater numbers and much harder than females. The dementias we know attack men in greater ratios include[16]:

- Parkinson's dementia (Lewy body dementia)
- Dementia with Lewy bodies (Lewy body dementia)
- Post-Stroke dementia (Vascular dementia)

- Multi-infarct dementia (Vascular dementia)
- Binswanger Disease(Vascular dementia)
- Normal pressure hydrocephalus
- Behavioral variant frontotemporal dementia
- Primary Progressive Aphasia (Frontotemporal dementia)
- Chronic traumatic encephalopathy
- HIV-related cognitive impairment
- Amyotrophic lateral sclerosis

From the data about the 19 primary dementias, at least eleven attack men in greater numbers. Data is not available for Creutzfeldt-Jakob disease, Wernicke-Korsakoff Syndrome, LATE, and Down syndrome with Alzheimer's disease. The remaining dementias strike both genders in similar numbers. When the authorities release more information, we will update this section.

If a minimum of 11 of 19 dementia types strike men in greater numbers than women, how can 68% of people living with dementia be women?

Alzheimer's accounts for 60-80% of dementia, and two-thirds of people with Alzheimer's are women.

When we say dementia attacks, women, 65% to 35% men, we distort the picture. I call on the medical community to provide greater clarity. More precise, we should warn women to represent two-thirds of total Alzheimer's cases, but stress a minimum of 11 of 19 dementia types strike men in greater numbers.

Treating dementia and Alzheimer's as interchangeable terms is misleading. There are 19 primary dementias and 11 or more attack men in greater numbers. If we exclude Alzheimer's and focus on the other 18 primary dementia types, they attack men by far greater percentages.

With that stipulation, let's explore why Alzheimer's and some dementias attack women more than men.

Why Does Alzheimer's & Dementia Strike Women in Greater Numbers Than Men?

In part, unique burdens & responsibilities explain the disparity.

Women still fight today for equality. Like Native Americans, African Americans, and African British, the average woman carries burdens; the average man is clueless.

To be a woman, one fights for equality from birth in a "man's world," as the song and tradition attest. Among things unique to women:

- Menstrual cycles (ranging from mild to horrendous)
- Childbirth
- Menopause

Being a guy is also difficult, but there's no denying women are born with unique responsibilities and burdens.

As an aunt once retorted, if they live long enough, every woman suffers menstrual cycles until menopause "tortures it out."

Women Live Longer

Women outlive men in the United States and worldwide.

Worldwide, the average man lives to age 69.8, while the average woman lives 74.2 years[17]. These are the average numbers, so they fluctuate from region to region and country to country.

Let's see how these numbers compare to the United States.

American Comparisons

The CDC reports the average American male lives 76 years, compared to the average American woman who lives 81 years[18].

Why Do Women Live Longer Than Men?

Although women live longer, this might result because

more men abuse alcohol, tobacco, and drugs, get less sleep, work in more hazardous jobs, suffer greater casualties in war, and take unnecessary risks.

The lead author of a study published in the *British Medical Journal*, Australian neuropsychiatrist Richard Cibulskis, confirmed some of my suspicions.

> *Men are much more likely to die from preventable and treatable non-communicable diseases, such as {ischemic} heart disease and lung cancer, and road traffic accidents*[19].

Global population expert, Dr. Perminder Sachdev, confirmed my other suspicions in an interview with *Time*.

"Men are more likely to smoke, drink excessively and be overweight," Sachdev said. "They are also less likely to seek medical help early, and, if diagnosed with a disease, they are more likely to be non-adherent to treatment." Sachdev also pointed out, "men are more likely to take life-threatening risks and to die in car accidents, brawls or gunfights[20]."

Although nature perhaps installed a natural order to preserve the female population, men's reckless nature might account for the five years difference in life expectancy between the genders.

It will interest to see if the numbers change as more women become more like men. Women are assuming greater roles in war, law enforcement, and other areas where even men with healthy habits have fallen. As the societal lines between men and women blur, the difference in life expectancy should fall.

In all honorable fields of life, women should go for it. Never has there been a better time to prove the equality of the sexes.

As far as men's bad habits, my hope is women continue to show better judgment and exercise greater restraint. Women will never prove their equality by emulating men's worse habits or trying to outdo us in the stupid department.

The best men and women rise on similar foundations. However, the worst men and women also share a foundation.

My hope for humans getting our act together soon hinges on the average woman being better than the average man.

Love yourselves for your unique feminine qualities. Be equal, but please do not confuse out-drinking, out-smoking, out-drugging, acting more reckless, and stupid than men with being equal. We need fewer men like that, not more women!

Chapter 4: DEMENTIA COSTS & PREVALENCE

In this chapter, we review dementia prevalence and costs to governments, the world, caregivers, and patients.

How Many People Worldwide Suffer Dementia?

According to the World Health Organization (WHO), over 50 million people suffer dementia worldwide, with 10 million new cases each year[21].

How Many Americans Have Dementia?

In the United States, 5.8 million Americans live with dementia[22], with Alzheimer's representing 70% of cases.

Let's check the UK dementia numbers.

How Many People In The UK Have Dementia?

According to the Alzheimer's Society, 850,000 people in the UK live with dementia[23].

Alzheimer's Society reports that about 70% of those living in UK care homes suffer dementia.

The numbers show Americans, British, and global citizens suffering high rates of dementia. Let's see which countries' dementia strikes the hardest.

Which Countries Have The Highest Dementia Rate?

Per World Atlas, the following ten countries suffer the highest dementia rate of deaths per 100,000 people[24]:

1. Finland
2. USA
3. Canada
4. Iceland
5. Sweden
6. Switzerland
7. Norway
8. Denmark
9. The Netherlands
10. Belgium

As we review the list, per population, dementia strikes Americans in greater numbers than any country but Finland.

Why?

There are several explanations:

- Over two-thirds of Americans are obese or overweight.
- The other countries on the list also suffer higher obesity levels than most countries not on the list.
- Because of weight issues, the countries in question suffer high rates of diabetes and high blood pressure, both dementia risk factors.
- Americans consume more prescription drugs than people worldwide. While there is no data to confirm, I suspect the other countries on the list also have greater access and use more prescription drugs than poorer countries.
- They load the western diet with salt, sugar, and

white processed flours.
- The average person in western countries lives longer than those in poorer nations.
- We will add other factors once data becomes available.
- People live longer in these countries than most not on the list (the older one lives, the greater the dementia risk)

Another explanation is more misdiagnosis and no-diagnosis in poorer countries around the world. Obesity and other risk factors are also less of a problem in developing countries.

I recommend global researchers compare the ten countries on this list. By viewing the similarities between the ten, we might better pinpoint the cause for Alzheimer's and the other dementias.

If we can figure out what the citizens from the ten nations are doing wrong, we can find the cause and means of preventing dementia. While I pointed to some of the most obvious risk factors, the most important common risk factor from the ten nations might be something unexpected.

Let's now examine dementia costs.

Dementia Costs

In this chapter, we analyze dementia costs. We examine the United States and global costs, then provide estimated costs per family.

What Does Dementia Cost the United States?

More than the entire economies of Finland and 166 other countries, dementia costs the United States $277 billion per year.

What Does Dementia Cost Worldwide?

Getting credible global numbers proves difficult, if not impossible, in any medical research. Often, the best source is the World Health Organization (WHO). They collect data from around the world and are an essential source for medical researchers.

Getting accurate dementia numbers in richer countries is difficult. In the United States and the UK, black people hesitate to take part in dementia studies or to seek medical attention for symptoms.

In richer countries, there are still too many misdiagnoses.

Thus, if we cannot get ironclad numbers in the United States, the United Kingdom, and the industrial nations, the task proves even more difficult for developing countries.

If the United States and the United Kingdom have difficulty convincing black citizens to seek medical attention for dementia symptoms, the third world faces even greater obstacles.

In the third world, most areas do well to offer their citizens basic medical care. With no urine or blood test, many regions lack resources for CAT scans, MRIs, and other expensive imaging equipment to make a diagnosis.

Without urine or blood tests, diagnosing dementia costs more than low-income people with inadequate or no insurance can afford in the richest countries.

In the United States and industrial nations, doctors often misdiagnose the other 19 primary dementias for Alzheimer's or each other.

Expecting doctors in many third world nations to diagnose dementia with inferior or no equipment is to expect miracles. If it overwhelms medical professionals in the wealthier nations, we often expect third world doctors to perform miracles. What amazes is they often do!

However, no matter how good a job the average third world doctor does treating typical medical conditions, even if trained, it does not equip them to diagnose dementia early, if at all. My comments are not criticism.

The average doctor's job is not to diagnose or treat dementia, but they must recognize symptoms and refer the patient to neurologists. Primary care physicians are the first line of defense.

North, south, east, west, dementia overwhelms the medical community.

Having discussed the limitations, let's examine the data. While the numbers are ballpark figures, landing in the park is the keystone to estimation. In most cases, the real numbers are much higher.

According to the *World Alzheimer's Report,* global dementia costs a minimum of $1 trillion per year, and experts predict it will reach $2 trillion by 2030 if we find no cure[25].

Authorities should release new numbers over the next year, and we will update this section.

The *Alzheimer's Report* global cost estimations do not include informal care costs; another reason we consider the estimates conservative.

The Alzheimer's Report concluded:

> *Direct medical care costs account for roughly 20% of global dementia costs, while direct social sector costs and informal care costs each account for roughly 40%. The relative contribution of informal care is greatest in the African regions and lowest in North America, Western Europe and some South American regions, while the reverse is true for social sector costs.*

Whatever the real up-to-date costs, we must take action to reduce the burden on individuals and nations. If we do not invest in independent research to develop an effective urine or blood test, cure, and vaccine for each dementia type, the costs will smother economies throughout the world. The costs will cripple developing countries and destabilize the wealthiest.

We have no choice but to invest more in dementia research. No matter which country you live, your economy, security, and the health of your nation rides on us finding a cure or vaccine.

As a scientist, I find it disturbing climate change and independent dementia research are not major priorities. Most governments, businesses, and individuals who can afford to fund dementia remain MIA in the war against dementia.

Before we conclude this section, let's examine the dementia statistics side-by-side in the table below.

EARLY-ONSET ALZHEIMER'S DISEASE (EOAD)

DEMENTIA STATISTICS

This table focuses on the number of people with dementia and the number of deaths per 100,000 among the nations chosen for comparison.

NATION	# OF PEOPLE WITH DEMENTIA	DEMENTIA DEATHS PER 100,000 PEOPLE	TOTAL COSTS (US DOLLARS)
Australia	447,115	29.61	$15 billion
Brazil	1 million +	10.71	$16.45 billion
Canadian	747,000	37.30	$10.4 billion
China	16.93 million	19.87	$69 billion
France	1.2 million	30.84	$37.91 billion
Germany	1.5 million	16.99	$57.57 billion
India	4 million	14.57	$28.38 billion
Italy	1.4 million	19.81	$29.96 billion
Japan	4.6 million	7.22	$14.8 billion
Mexico	800,000	3.62	Not available
Spain	800.000+	29.23	$19.98 million
Netherlands	280,000	39.37	$4.44 million
United States	5.8 million	44.41	$290 billion
United Kingdom	850,000	49.18	$26.3 billion

Sources: World Health Rankings[26], Alzheimer's Europe[27], NATSIM[28], Alzheimer's Society[29], Brain Test[30]

Other sources cited in the chapter.

The table comes from my book <u>2020 Dementia Overview</u>, which covers cost and prevalence among comparative nations in greater detail.

Let's next discuss the dementia costs for caregivers.

What Does Dementia Cost Volunteer Caregivers?

Although 41% make less than $50,000, American voluntary caregivers devote a minimum of 18.4 billion hours per year to dementia patients.

Worth $232 billion per year, we underrate the voluntary caregiving heroes in our fight against dementia. This total does not include lost wages for the voluntary caregiver.

According to the Northwestern Mutual C.A.R.E. Study, 67% of voluntary caregivers must cut their living to help pay for the patient's medical care, and 57% end up experiencing financial problems[31].

Adding to the costs of voluntary caregivers, they often end up sick themselves. Caring for loved ones with dementia bankrupts many.

In the early stages, the loved one can still perform most of their daily tasks but will require 24/7 care once the symptoms advance.

Imagine putting your life on hold for years to care, bathe, feed, protect, and take such a heavy load on your shoulders.

Millions of dementia families face the dilemma where the husband and wife both must work in most families to get by. You work as a couple to build stability in your own family, and then, boom, doctors diagnose one of you with dementia.

What Does Dementia Cost Dementia Patients?

When we say patient, past a certain stage in the disease, we refer to family or loved ones. A person who cannot perform daily tasks cannot manage finances, even if they have any left.

Too often, the costs drive entire families into bankruptcy because of dementia costs for a member.

Authorities estimate the average cost per dementia patient is $341,840, with families expected to cover 70 percent.

The costs devastate the average family in the industrial nations.

How are they supposed to afford it in developing countries where the average citizen makes less than one-thousand American dollars per year?

Dementia Recap

Although your dementia research has just begun, you now have a decent overview of Dementia.

In Chapter One, we explored dementia. We turned to several top dementia or medical organizations and compared their definitions.

Chapter two explained Alzheimer's is to dementia what China is to Asia. We listed the 19 dementias. They include:

1. Dementia with Lewy Bodies
2. Parkinson's Disease Dementia
3. Corticobasal Syndrome
4. Typical Alzheimer's Disease
5. Posterior Cortical Atrophy
6. Down Syndrome with Alzheimer's
7. Limbic-predominant Age-related TDP-43 Encephalopathy (LATE)
8. Early-onset Alzheimer's
9. Behavioral Variant Frontotemporal Dementia
10. Progressive Supranuclear Palsy
11. Nonfluent Primary Progressive Aphasia
12. Logopenic Progressive Aphasia
13. Cortical Vascular Dementia
14. Binswanger Disease
15. Normal Pressure Hydrocephalus
16. Huntington's Disease
17. Korsakoff Syndrome
18. Creutzfeldt-Jakob Disease
19. Amyotrophic Lateral Sclerosis

Although most the dementia types share similar symptoms, enough to cause misdiagnosis, each has its unique pathology and symptoms.

In chapter three, we explored dementia prevalence in the United States, the UK, and worldwide.

Chapter four examined who is most likely to get dementia. We found Native Americans (those who greeted the first Europeans), and black citizens in the United States and the UK are more likely to get dementia than their white or Asian counterparts.

We also explored the women to men ratio. Women represent two-thirds of Alzheimer's and over sixty percent of dementia cases. We pointed out the Alzheimer's figure skews the dementia numbers because men are more likely to get a minimum of 11 of the 19 primary dementia types.

Chapter four explored the US, UK, global, patient, family, and voluntary caregivers' dementia costs. The staggering numbers are almost as frightening as the medical disorder itself.

We borrowed the following table from *2020 Dementia Overview*.

Dementia Costs & Prevalence

NATION	# OF PEOPLE WITH DEMENTIA	DEMENTIA DEATHS PER 100,000 PEOPLE	TOTAL COSTS (US DOLLARS)
Australia	447,115	29.61	$15 billion
Brazil	1 million +	10.71	$16.45 billion
Canadian	747,000	37.30	$10.4 billion
China	16.93 million	19.87	$69 billion
France	1.2 million	30.84	$37.91 billion
Germany	1.5 million	16.99	$57.57 billion
India	4 million	14.57	$28.38 billion
Italy	1.4 million	19.81	$29.96 billion
Japan	4.6 million	7.22	$14.8 billion
Mexico	800,000	3.62	Not available
Spain	800.000+	29.23	$19.98 million
Netherlands	280,000	39.37	$4.44 million
United States	5.8 million	44.41	$290 billion
United Kingdom	850,000	49.18	$26.3 billion

Sources: World Health Rankings[32], Alzheimer's Europe[33], NATSIM[34], Alzheimer's Society[35], Brain Test[36]

The table comes from <u>2020 Dementia Overview</u>, which covers cost and prevalence among comparative nations in greater detail.

After reviewing the conservative numbers, and factoring in an aging population, we concluded we must find a cure before it

EARLY-ONSET ALZHEIMER'S DISEASE (EOAD)

bankrupts millions of families and cripples nations.

Having explained the series and introduced dementia, let's discuss the 19 primary dementia types.

Chapter 5: 19 PRIMARY DEMENTIA TYPES

Why is it important to learn about the most prevalent dementias?

There are several reasons. One, the dementias share similar symptoms and—with no accurate testing—doctors often misdiagnose for one of a hundred or more other possibilities. Two, if a person gets one dementia, more often than not, they develop an overlapping second dementia type, known as mixed dementia. In some cases, three dementia types might develop in later stages.

The pathology, related-proteins, atrophy location, and the resulting symptoms determine dementia classifications.

The more we learn about dementia, dementia types, and subtypes grow.

We once thought of Alzheimer's disease as one sweeping neurological disorder, but now know there is typical Alzheimer's, behavior variant Alzheimer's, posterior cortical atrophy, Early-onset Alzheimer's, and the newest dementia category, LATE, previously misdiagnosed for typical Alzheimer's. If that is not complicated enough, there are 20-40 typical Alzheimer's types.

Depending on the pathology, the three primary progressive aphasia subtypes are either Alzheimer's or frontotemporal-related.

We know there is not one vascular dementia, but three: post-stroke dementia, multi-infarct dementia, and Binswanger disease.

There are two Lewy body dementias; Parkinson's disease dementia and dementia with Lewy bodies. There are also other Parkinson-related neurological disorders.

The series covers the 19 most prevalent dementia types. As noted, several are subtypes, but this work extends each equal status and inquiry

Besides breaking down the twenty most prevalent dementia types, we also discuss subtypes for each.

To reduce repetition, we divide the 19 dementias into the following sections.

Lewy Body/Parkinsonism Related Dementias

1. *Dementia with Lewy Bodies*
2. *Parkinson's Disease Dementia*
3. Corticobasal Syndrome

Alzheimer's Related Dementias

4. Typical Alzheimer's Disease
5. *Posterior Cortical Atrophy*
6. *Down Syndrome with Alzheimer's*
7. *Limbic-predominant Age-related TDP-43 Encephalopathy (LATE)*
8. Early-onset Alzheimer's

Frontotemporal Lobar Degeneration Related Dementias

9. *Behavioral Variant Frontotemporal Dementia*
10. Progressive Supranuclear Palsy

Primary Progressive Aphasia Related Dementias

11. *Nonfluent Primary Progressive Aphasia (nfvPPA)*
12. Logopenic Progressive Aphasia (LPA)

Vascular Dementia

13. *Cortical Vascular Dementia*
14. *Binswanger Disease*

Other Dementias

15. *Normal Pressure Hydrocephalus*
16. *Huntington's Disease*
17. *Korsakoff Syndrome*
18. *Creutzfeldt-Jakob Disease*
19. Amyotrophic Lateral Sclerosis

II. EARLY-ONSET ALZHEIMER'S DISEASE (EOAD) DEMENTIAS

Let's shift the focus to the book's topic, early-onset Alzheimer's disease (EOAD).

Only age makes EOAD a dementia classification, for if it did not strike younger people, there would be no reason for a separate distinction.

For this book, unless specified, whether I use the terms early-onset Alzheimer's disease, EOAD, Alzheimer's, AD, we are discussing EOAD.

Chapter 6: WHAT IS ALZHEIMER'S DISEASE?

Alzheimer's is an "irreversible, progressive brain disorder," according to the National Institute on Aging[37], "that slowly destroys memory and thinking skills, and, eventually, the ability to carry out the simplest tasks."

Alzheimer's disease accounts for sixty to eighty percent of all dementia. Scientists don't know the exact numbers because doctors often misdiagnose the different dementias for each other. Adding to the confusion, Alzheimer's is often present with other types of dementias[38].

A minimum of twenty percent of people suffering from other forms of dementia also end up with Alzheimer's. It's one of the most prevalent, devastating, and cruel diseases of our day.

Who Discovered Alzheimer's Disease?

In 1906, Dr. Alois Alzheimer discovered Alzheimer's when studying the brain of a woman who suffered cognitive decline, erratic behavior, and a diminished ability to communicate in the years, leading to her death. Before Dr. Alzheimer's discovery, the medical world and families lumped Alzheimer's patients into the "crazy" or "lost their mind" category. Most of the world is only now learning what Dr. Alzheimer knew in 1906.

The disease blindsides the average family when it strikes a member.

As difficult as the disease remains today, one can only imagine the indignities and horrors victims suffered before Dr. Alzheimer's discovery.

Alzheimer's Canada explains the discovery.

> *Dr. Alois Alzheimer first identified the disease in 1906. He described the two hallmarks of the disease: 'plaques,' which are numerous tiny, dense deposits scattered throughout the*

> *brain that become toxic to brain cells at excessive levels, and 'tangles,' which interfere with vital processes, eventually choking off the living cells. When brain cells degenerate and die, the brain markedly shrinks in some regions[39].*

Dr. Alzheimer discovered entangled lumps of fiber now called tau (neurofibrillary or tangles), and unusual clusters on the woman's brain since named amyloid plaques.

Other Alzheimer's Definitions

Let's turn to some respected authorities and see how they define Alzheimer's.

Alzheimer's Association

The Alzheimer's Association defines Alzheimer's:

> *Alzheimer's is a type of dementia that causes problems with memory, thinking, and behavior. Symptoms usually develop and get worse over time, becoming severe enough to interfere with daily tasks[40].*

What to take from the quote: Alzheimer's causes memory deficits and erratic behavior. While symptoms develop slow, Alzheimer's becomes debilitating in later stages.

Mayo Clinic

Let's review the Mayo Clinic's definition: [41]

> *Alzheimer's disease is a progressive disease that destroys memory and other important mental functions. At first, someone with Alzheimer's disease may notice mild confusion and difficulty remembering. Eventually, people with the disease may even forget important people in their lives and undergo dramatic personality changes.*

What to take from the quote: The Mayo Clinic affirms the

Alzheimer's Association's definition.

UK Alzheimer's Society

Let's turn to the UK and review how the Alzheimer's Society defines Alzheimer's[42]:

> *Alzheimer's disease is the most common cause of dementia. The word dementia describes a set of symptoms that can include memory loss and difficulties with thinking, problem-solving, or language. These symptoms occur when the brain is damaged by certain diseases, including Alzheimer's disease.*

What to take from the quote: The Alzheimer's Society confirms Alzheimer's disease causes memory loss and inhibits one's ability to communicate and solve problems.

Every day (normal), life becomes more difficult as the disease progresses.

Alzheimer's disease attacks the brain and destroys one's personality, much as rampaging barbarians who pillage a village until it is no more.

Since there is no cure, there are only three things we can do regarding Alzheimer's:

1. Adopt a lifestyle to slow or prevent Alzheimer's.
2. Continue the search for a cure.
3. Ease the burden on victims and their loved ones.

In stage one, Alzheimer's shows no symptoms.

An Alzheimer's diagnosis shocks, but there is no time to waste. Now is the time to live like there might not be a tomorrow. We cover this more in-depth in the sections on diagnosis and stages.

Besides preparing for the future, embrace the earlier stages of the disease and squeeze as much quality time as possible. This stage is the last ride of normalcy, so make the most of it.

What is Alzheimer's relationship to dementia?

Let's next review Alzheimer's relationship with dementia.

Much like China is one country within Asia, Alzheimer's is one dementia. As China is the largest country within Asia, Alzheimer's is the most prevalent dementia.

The different dementias share many symptoms, often causing misdiagnosis.

Adding to the confusion, doctors cannot confirm it is Alzheimer's until one dies, and they perform an autopsy. We need tests to detect different dementias, including Alzheimer's.

Plaques, Neurofibrillary Tangles, Communication Breakdown

When studying Alzheimer's, the terms *amyloid plaques, neurofibrillary tangles,* and *loss connection* appear because they are the markers of the disease. Let's examine each, starting with amyloid plaques.

Amyloid Plaques

Beta-amyloid is a single-molecule protein that forms plaques in the brain and clumps into amyloid plaques. The toxic plaque grows and disrupts the synapses connecting the brain's neurons.

The amyloid plaques form in the brains of people who do not have Alzheimer's, but the clumps are smaller. Those with Alzheimer's have a higher concentration of the plaque and in the hippocampus area of the brain responsible for emotions, learning, and memory.

Stanford University School of Medicine Study

A team of Stanford and Harvard scientists investigated how beta-amyloid elevates the risk of Alzheimer's. Carla Shatz, Ph.D., professor of neurobiology and biology and senior author of the study, shared their results.

"Our discovery," said Shatz, "suggests that Alzheimer's disease starts to manifest long before plaque formation becomes evident." Shatz also reported[43]:

> *Beta-amyloid begins life as a solitary molecule but tends to bunch up — initially into small clusters that are still soluble and can travel freely in the brain, and finally into the plaques that are hallmarks of Alzheimer's. The study showed for the first time that in this clustered form, beta-amyloid can bind strongly to a receptor on nerve cells, setting in motion an intercellular process that erodes their synapses with other nerve cells.*

Such discoveries add one more layer to the challenge but get us a step closer to understanding what causes Alzheimer's, so we can find a cure. Science is conducting and analyzing tests to determine why amyloid plaques develop and how to prevent them from damaging neurons.

We next study Neurofibrillary Tangles.

Neurofibrillary Tangles

What Dr. Alzheimer referred to as "tangled bundles of fiber," now called neurofibrillary tangles, are uncommon levels of the tau protein that form inside neurons.

Normal tau protein protects neurons, but abnormal or muted versions accumulate inside and kill neurons, which creates Alzheimer's symptoms, including abnormal behavior, memory loss, inability to organize, and plan.

Why are tangles and plaques a problem? Before we move on, let's examine how the brain functions and how the tangles and plaques cause problems.

Loss of Connection

The plaques and tangles break the connections (synapses) between the brain's neurons (nerve cells). When this happens, the brain functions much like an electronic device with a short in the wires. If the neurons are unconnected, the brain cannot send messages to other brain parts, muscles, and organs within the body[44].

Neurons

In a neuron forest, close to 100 trillion branches connect about 100 billion nerve cells in the brain and nervous system. This vast communication network allows the different parts of the brain to function and us to direct our body parts.

When the neurons cannot transmit messages, the affected parts of the brain, and body breakdown, arms will not move unless the brain commands, and the same is true from head to toe.

Alzheimer's attacks the hippocampus area of the brain, the part that stores and processes memory, but spreads to other areas of the brain as Alzheimer's develops.

A fatal disease that kills and has no cure is cruel because Alzheimer's moves in methodical steps to block the connection between neurons, and removes one's memory, reasoning skills, thinking ability, recognition skills, and in advance-stages attacks motor skills and organs.

Communication is a key component of life, and much is going on behind the scenes we are oblivious. When Alzheimer's destroys the neurons' ability to communicate, everything that is us disappears.

Science is still probing to find what causes amyloid plaques and neurofibrillary tangles, but one group of scientists believe they have found a vaccination to block both the amyloid plaques and neurofibrillary tangles from growing.

University of Texas (UT) Southwestern Medical Center Develop Alzheimer's Vaccine

Unsuccessful until now, the researchers at the UT Southwestern Medical Center developed a vaccine to "arm the body to attack Alzheimer's plaques and tangles before they even start to shut down the brain[45]."

Scientists have conducted extensive and successful tests on mice. While such tests on animals do not always work on humans, the results remain promising, and scientists will push forward.

Director of the UT Southwestern Alzheimer's Disease Center, Dr. Roger Rosenbert explained the potential breakthrough[46]:

> *The significance of these findings is that DNA Aβ42 trimer immunotherapy targets two major pathologies in AD – amyloid plaques and neurofibrillary tangles – in one vaccine without inducing inflammatory T-cell responses, which carry the danger of autoimmune inflammation, as found in a clinical trial using active Aβ42 peptide immunization in patients with AD {Alzheimer's}.*

It is a lengthy process to test humans and get FDA approval, but we hope they soon develop vaccines to spare most people from Alzheimer's and the other dementias.

What Age Do Alzheimer's Symptoms First Occur?

There are two versions of Alzheimer's, young or early-onset Alzheimer's and regular Alzheimer's, the former rare and genetic, the latter prevalent and science suggests caused by nongenetic factors.

The primary difference between the two is early-onset strikes younger people, in their forties and fifties.

Young Or Early-Onset Alzheimer's

Young or early-onset Alzheimer's attacks people in their forties and fifties[47]. The medical community estimates 200,000 Americans have early-onset Alzheimer's[48].

Almost identical symptoms as normal Alzheimer's, early-onset Alzheimer's hits people decades before the regular version strikes.

According to Johns Hopkins Medicine, most people with early-onset Alzheimer's have the common version, but a few hundred have Genetic (familial) Alzheimer's disease. Those with these rare genes experience symptoms as early as age thirty[49].

Regular Alzheimer's

There is a reason many refer to Alzheimer's as the "old folks disease." The first signs appear in a person's mid-sixties[50].

How Many People Suffer Alzheimer's Disease?

In this section, we will investigate how many people suffer Alzheimer's in the United States and worldwide. Officials believe the actual numbers are much higher.

Because of inadequate health systems in the third world and difficulties diagnosing Alzheimer's (no accurate test) worldwide, all we know for certain is the numbers are worse than we can verify.

"Some people with the disease never receive a diagnosis," said officials at the National Institute on Aging. "Many others have dementia-related conditions, such as aspiration pneumonia, listed as the primary cause of death while the underlying cause, Alzheimer's, is never reported[51]."

Despite the limited data, enough death certificates list Alzheimer's as a cause of death to make the disease the sixth leading killer in the United States.

Authorities compute the numbers from death certificates and scientific studies, which causes them to underestimate the total. You could add ten or twenty percent and perhaps reach a closer number, but we use the more conservative official numbers for this discussion.

First, we will focus on the United States numbers, then examine global numbers.

How Many Alzheimer's Cases Are There In The United States?

With one new case every 65 seconds[52], 5.7 million Americans[53] live with Alzheimer's.

How many Americans die from Alzheimer's?

In 2014, the last time they updated their numbers, the CDC attributed 93,500 American deaths to Alzheimer's disease[54].

These are the latest numbers. When officials release more recent official figures, we will update this section. The updated numbers should be much higher as the number of people with Alzheimer's has continued to rise.

More Americans die from Alzheimer's than heart disease, breast cancer, and prostate cancer totaled[55].

We Need A Better System

In the computer age, officials should enter death certificates into a national pool with a cause of death, a copy of the birth certificate, and any related disease such as Alzheimer's, cancer, diabetes, or any other ailment that perhaps caused the pneumonia or whatever listed as the cause of death on the certificates.

It seems everybody in the world has our information except those who need it to do good. A national computer network would provide instant updates on the causes of death and help achieve more accurate information.

Such a system would arm medical researchers with more accurate and updated information, doctors with more weapons to diagnose and treat diseases, and patients with a better chance of recovery.

Instead of trailing other industrial countries, the United

States must develop a quality health care system, the rest of the world wants to copy. The current disastrous American and global health systems of diagnosing, treating, and reporting are insufficient.

How many Alzheimer's cases are there in the world?

There is a new case of dementia, the majority Alzheimer's, every 3 seconds[56]. Authorities diagnose almost 10 million people each year, and 50 million people live with the disease worldwide[57].

How many humans die each year from Alzheimer's?

Getting an exact number of Alzheimer's deaths in the United States is difficult because death certificates often list pneumonia or some associated disease as the cause of death. Worldwide, the job is impossible.

The World Alzheimer's Report 2018 illustrates the problem and calls every nation to step forward to meet the challenge:

> *Many countries have no diagnostic tools, no access to clinical trials and, indeed, few, if any, specialized doctors and researchers. Where those are present they may not have the means to travel and to communicate their ideas. Yet, with the biggest increases in dementia occurring in LMICs, does this make sense? Shouldn't the governments of those countries try to contribute to research for the benefit of their populations rather than relying on other countries, such as the USA and the UK, to lead the way[58]?*

The suggestion is easier said than done in countries already struggling to keep their heads above water. The words seem somewhat harsh, considering how impoverished the poorest countries are, but as we will soon address, costs threaten to bury even the largest and richest nations.

Every three seconds, somebody in the world gets Alzheimer's or one of the other dementias.

There are 50 million global cases of dementia. Because of misdiagnosis and reporting issues, this number is likely much higher.

How many people worldwide die from Alzheimer's?

Worldwide, dementia—Alzheimer's, representing 60 to 80 percent—is the fourth leading cause of death, totaling 2.38 million[59].

Dementia (Alzheimer's) kills more people than:

- Lower respiratory infections
- Neonatal deaths
- Diarrheal diseases
- Road incidents
- Liver disease
- Tuberculosis
- Kidney disease
- Digestive disease
- HIV/AIDS
- Suicide
- Malaria
- Homicide
- Nutritional deficiencies
- Meningitis
- Protein-energy malnutrition
- Drowning
- Maternal deaths
- Parkinson's disease
- Alcohol disorder
- Intestinal infectious diseases
- Drug disorder
- Hepatitis
- Fire

- Conflict
- Heat or cold-related deaths
- Terrorism
- Natural disasters

Alzheimer's and the dementias kill more people than every other disease except for cardiovascular disease, cancers, and respiratory disease.

While the official numbers are staggering, we know the total as Alzheimer's and dementia numbers are low because authorities often list pneumonia or other dementia symptoms as the cause of death.

To American and Global Government and Medical Officials

Beller Health calls on the governments and medical communities of the world to step to the plate and provide researchers instant, detailed information about the cause of death, other health conditions, and other invaluable health data.

There are privacy and legal issues to work through, but there is too much avoidable human death and suffering because researchers too often are estimating what medical records should make crystal clear.

If privacy issues mean blackout names, addresses, and other personal information, do it. The information people want to protect is unnecessary. Researchers need age, cause of death, medical history, notes of importance for medical research.

Help save and enhance lives by providing accurate information!

Does Alzheimer's Discriminate?

We investigated whether Alzheimer's discriminates against any groups. What we found is the disease discriminates against:

Elderly

The greatest Alzheimer's risk factor is age[60].

Females

Although science is uncertain why women represent two-thirds of Alzheimer's patients[61].

African Americans

African Americans are two to three times as likely, as whites, to get Alzheimer's[62].

Diabetes and high blood sugar

Several studies suggest diabetes and high blood sugar elevates the risk of Alzheimer's[63].

Down syndrome

People with down syndrome have a 50-50 chance of getting Alzheimer's[64].

High blood pressure

Higher blood pressure increases the risk of Alzheimer's[65].

Inactive minds

Inactive minds increase the chance of Alzheimer's. The brain needs exercise, too[66].

Obesity

Being overweight raises Alzheimer's risk[67].

Physical inactivity

Physical inactivity is dangerous and elevates the risk of Alzheimer's[68].

Unhealthy diets

Nobody can do anything about being elderly, female, African American, or if they have down syndrome. A healthier lifestyle, however, will help us avoid obesity, inactive minds, lack of exercise, diabetes, and high blood pressure. Besides the higher risks to other diseases, the Alzheimer's numbers should wake us all up to how important it is to feed and exercise our bodies and minds.

Of the list, two stand out and require closer examination: females and African Americans.

Do Women Have A Higher Risk Of Alzheimer's?

While Alzheimer's does not discriminate by race, the disease strikes older people and females in disproportionate numbers. The higher number of females is in part because they outlive males.

United States

The life expectancy in the United States ranks 53 out of 100 nations where such statistics exist. The average American male lives 76.99 years, and females 81.88 years[69].

United Kingdom

In the UK, Alzheimer's and the other dementias kill more women than any other single cause of death[70]. Also, of all UK Alzheimer's and dementia cases, 61 percent are female and only 39 percent men[71].

Worldwide

Women are 2.5 times more likely than men to get Alzheimer's[72]. According to the World Health Organization, Alzheimer's is the fifth leading global cause of death for women[73].

In the US, the UK, and worldwide, Alzheimer's and the dementias strike women harder than men.

Let's review the numbers for African Americans.

Do African Americans Have A Higher Risk Of Alzheimer's?

United States

According to one analysis of dozens of studies, the researchers concluded African Americans are underrepresented, and more unwilling to take part[74].

This reluctance might result from historical abuses such as the Tuskegee experiments. Whatever the reason, scientists and researchers must earn this trust, and African Americans must take part in studies for science to figure out what causes the higher ratio of Alzheimer's among the African American population.

Victimized in the past by systematic bigotry, African Americans fear unfair treatment if diagnosed with Alzheimer's.

Let's review the UK and global numbers to determine if the trend is exclusive American.

United Kingdom

Black British citizens are at a higher risk of Alzheimer's and other dementias than are their white or Asian counterparts. A group of researchers studied 2.5 million people.

The study found black women were 25 percent more likely to suffer Alzheimer's or dementia than white women, and black men 28 percent more likely than white men[75].

One of the leading authors, Dr. Tra My Pham, of UCL's Institute of Epidemiology and Health, explained their findings.

"What we found suggests that the rates of people receiving a diagnosis may be lower than the actual rates of dementia in certain groups, among black men," Pham said. "It is concerning that black people appear to be more at risk of dementia but less likely to receive a timely diagnosis[76]."

Science does not know the exact cause for the higher rates, but the study's lead author, Dr. Claudia Cooper, offered insight. "Our new findings may reflect, for example, that there are inequalities in the care people receive to prevent and treat illnesses associated with dementia," said Cooper. "Or perhaps GPs or patients' families are reluctant to name dementia in communities where more stigma is associated with a dementia diagnosis[77]."

We see a similar pattern in the US and UK. Are these consistent with global trends? It is impossible to say, for we could not find any credible data. We hope new data will shed new light on the subject, which we add in the next annual edition.

What we have learned is Alzheimer's and the dementias attack all groups of people, but strike women and blacks harder than whites and Asians.

Based on known Alzheimer's risks, what combination would make the perfect Alzheimer's candidate?

Perfect Alzheimer's Candidate

An overweight, 65-year-old African American female who does not exercise, eats unhealthy, has high blood pressure and diabetes, does not challenge her mind, and suffers down syndrome would be the perfect candidate for Alzheimer's. She would carry ten high-risk factors, four out of her control, and six within.

Like everybody else, women and blacks need to view the risk factors under their control. While a few factors are beyond our best efforts, every human must develop better habits for the components we govern. And, all people must demand more from the authorities in funding impartial studies for accurate tests, cures, and better treatment for a disease that destroys the golden years for over a third of humans fortunate to make it to their sixties.

Next, we will review the financial costs of Alzheimer's.

How Much Does Alzheimer's Cost?

No thorough discussion about Alzheimer's can exclude financial costs. If we do not find a cure or cheaper, better treatment for this disease, it will bankrupt most countries by 2050. The individual and government costs are already reaching unbearable levels.

We will break the costs into four categories:

1. Individual
2. United States
3. Global
4. Volunteer caregivers

Although enormous, this section does not focus on human costs. While we emphasize the financial hardships, at no time are we implying the financial costs are greater than the horror those carrying the disease must endear, nor the difficulties caregivers face.

Let's review the individual costs before discussing the national and global costs, and the estimated financial hardship on voluntary caregivers.

Individual Costs

Besides the human suffering by the patient and families, the costs for treating one person with Alzheimer's is a minimum of $424,000, and this does not include the costs to a family in lost wages[78].

Families around the world make difficult decisions when one member suffers Alzheimer's/dementia. A stable middle-class family can fall through the cracks.

Profit motives and other factors price medical care for diseases like Alzheimer's out of the reach of most Americans and global citizens, who have modest incomes, bad or no health insurance

United States Alzheimer's Prevalence

5.8 million Americans suffer Alzheimer's, and the total will grow to 13.8 million[79] by 2050. To add weight to the number, the number of Americans who have Alzheimer's or dementia exceeds the population of 46 states[80].

The officials are dropping the ball because they remain inactive against the greatest human disaster and financial crisis facing Americans and the government.

Please study the chart below to gauge Alzheimer's costs now and the future.

YEAR	US ALZHEIMER'S CASES	COST
2018	5.8 million	$277 million
2050	13.8 million	$1.1 trillion

The numbers come from BrainTest[81], Forbes[82], Alzheimer's Impact Movement[83], Bright Focus Foundation[84], Alzheimer's Association's annual Alzheimer's Disease Facts and Figures[85].

Please note reality is much worse than the numbers above, which do not include the misdiagnosed cases or the Americans walking around with dementia and do not know.

According to the Bright Light Foundation, over 500,000 Americans die from Alzheimer's disease each year.

Alzheimer's and the dementias are an epidemic and threaten the financial security of the nation and American families. The dementia cost wipes out savings and bankrupt families, and the burden dumped on taxpayers is growing insurmountable. Like our health system, something must give on costs.

United States Costs

As a nation, Americans spent a minimum of $277 billion in 2018 and will surpass $1.1 trillion by 2050, unless we win the war against Alzheimer's and the dementias[86].

The Alzheimer's Association reports:

> This {2018 costs} is approximately 48 percent of the net value of Walmart sales in 2017 ($481.3 billion) and nine times the total revenue of McDonald's in 2016 ($24.6 billion).

When politicians talk about waste, they should be ashamed for not investing more in finding accurate testing and a cure for Alzheimer's. Americans suffer on the level of continuous long term torture, and the costs are bankrupting families and our health care system, but politicians are MIA in a real war.

Let's review the global costs.

Global Altheimer's

Across the globe, the disease is no less devastating. Many international medical authorities, misdiagnose, under-treat, and under-report Alzheimer's.

Global Cases

According to the Bright Focus Foundation, by 2050, there will be a minimum of 152 million people who have Alzheimer's or another dementia[87].

Entering 2020, over 50 million people fight Alzheimer's/dementia.

The 2019 Alzheimer's cases exceed the entire population of 187 of 195 countries[88] in the world[89]. Since the numbers are under-reported, the situation is even worse. Yet there is no coordinated effort between governments to defeat this global epidemic.

Other than climate change, there is no greater threat to humans and the global financial market than Alzheimer's and the other dementias.

What is the estimated world costs?

Global costs related to Alzheimer's and dementia will be a minimum of $1 Trillion in 2019 and will double by 2030, if not before.

Like the United States, international human and financial costs are overwhelming families and governments.

Please review the Alzheimer's/dementia global costs in the table below.

YEAR	GLOBAL ALZHEIMER'S CASES	COST
2018	50 million	$1 trillion
2050	152 million	$9.12 trillion

The costs are from a study released in the Journal of the Alzheimer's Association[90].

The reported United States and global numbers are low. As people age from and become the largest living generation, these costs will become unbearable for the younger generations.

Alzheimer's and dementia destroys individuals, families, and countries. Preventing Alzheimer's and the other dementias should be in the top three priorities of every nation in the world.

Volunteer Caregivers

Alzheimer's is a 24/7 job in the later stages, and much of this burden falls on volunteer caregivers. Besides the horrors for Alzheimer's patients, volunteer caregivers suffer great financial loss, depression, stress, often resulting in health issues.

Over 16.1 million Americans provide 18.4 billion hours of volunteer care worth $232 billion to people carrying Alzheimer's and the dementias[91].

As you can see, Americans devote an enormous amount of needed care to loved ones suffering from Alzheimer's. The figures only account for what it would cost to hire somebody to do the work of volunteers and does not include the enormous amount of lost wages.

Other than those suffering Alzheimer's, nobody carries a bigger burden than those who offer invaluable voluntary care.

We will next face one of Alzheimer's frustrating realities.

What Causes Alzheimer's?

Whatever causes Alzheimer's disease deserves a chapter, but science offers little but a hypothesis and preliminary tests on lab animals. Until they find a breakthrough, this chapter remains incomplete.

For decades, the world's top neurologists have failed to determine Alzheimer's exact cause. Not knowing the cause, all Alzheimer's drug trials fail.

Discovering the cause (s) should provide researchers the information they need to develop accurate tests for Alzheimer's like they do cardiovascular and other diseases.

Researchers and the medical community uncovered several risk factors, but no cure.

Section four probes the risks, which provide clues about how to prevent or slow the disease.

For now, that is the best science offers.

We hope researchers soon give us a reason to rewrite this chapter and describe the exact cause (s) of Alzheimer's disease.

We debated whether to include this chapter and did so to emphasize the importance. The elusive cause is essential to finding a cure. Therefore, this chapter remains incomplete.

Let's examine Alzheimer's symptoms.

Alzheimer's Subtypes

Complicating efforts to cure Alzheimer's, evidence shows there is not one Alzheimer's but a minimum three.

Several researchers and neurologists pointed towards Alzheimer's variances for decades, arguing one size does not fit all cases. The argument picked up steam in 2015 after back-to-back studies confirmed what neurologists long observed.

A two-year study released in 2015 by UCLA built on a smaller study and determined there is not one Alzheimer's, but at least three versions. The study's lead author, Dr. Dale Bredesen, a UCLA professor of neurology and distinguished neurodegenerative disease researcher, led the team.

"Because the presentation varies from person to person, there has been suspicion for years that Alzheimer's represents more than one illness," said Bredesen. "When laboratory tests go beyond the usual tests, we find these three distinct subtypes[92]."

In 2020, we believe there are three Alzheimer's subtypes:

1. Typical Alzheimer's
2. Posterior Cortical Atrophy (pre-dominant posterior atrophy or Benson's syndrome or parietal-dominant atrophy)
3. LATE (Limbic-predominant age-related TDP-43) or Medial Temporal Atrophy

Every piece we find in the Alzheimer's and dementia puzzle reminds us how little we know overall. In part explaining why a cure remains beyond our reach, each subtype causes different symptoms and require different cures.

Most drug trials and research focus on Alzheimer's as a singular disorder, but the subtypes explain, in part, why all drug trials have ended in failure. There will not be one cure, but by discovering the subtypes, we might discover a cure for each.

A breakthrough in treating cancer provided hope to those who suffer or treat Alzheimer's and dementia. When researchers sequenced tumor genomes and compared them to patients' genomes to develop a methodical and exact treatment plan, those interested in an Alzheimer's cure took notice. Dementia patients and doctors hoped modern medicine could do the same with Alzheimer's disease.

In Alzheimer's, however, there is no such tumor or biopsy markers like cancer. How did the UCLA team overcome this obstacle?

"So how do we get an idea about what is driving the process?" said Bredesen. "The approach we took was to use the underlying metabolic mechanisms of the disease process to guide the establishment of an extensive set of laboratory tests, such as fasting insulin, copper-to-zinc ratio, and dozens of others."

Researchers identify over 100 disorders leading to dementia. While we focus on the 19, causing 99% of dementia cases, the fact remains there are over 100 dementia subtypes. When science figures out more of the Alzheimer's puzzle, there might be a dozen or more subtypes.

Our focus in this book is typical Alzheimer's disease, and we devote a book to each, but let's discuss each subtype first.

Three Alzheimer's Types

According to neurologist Dale Bredesen, Alzheimer's results from 1) inflammation, 2) inadequate nutrient levels, and 3) "other synapse-supporting molecules, and exposures." By separating Alzheimer's into three subtypes, Bredesen and other researchers found different treatments for each.

Instead of viewing amyloid plaque deposits as the cause, Bredesen and other neurologists consider the deposits the amyloid protein's effort to protect the brain from true Alzheimer's causes. These neurologists point to the wide range of Alzheimer's risk factors and diverse pathology to suggest there is not one Alzheimer's but four.

1. Inflammatory (Typical Alzheimer's)
2. Posterior Cortical Atrophy (Cortical)
3. Limbic-predominant age-related TDP-43 encephalopathy (LATE)
4. Early-onset Alzheimer's disease

LATE represents a significant number of older people before misdiagnosed for typical Alzheimer's. Depending on how science proceeds, LATE is either an Alzheimer's subtype or an Alzheimer's-like dementia.

For this book, we link the subtypes to Alzheimer's, but also cover them as distinctive dementia types. While typical Alzheimer's remains the most prevalent, the other three subtypes combined total of almost fifty percent of Alzheimer's cases, making each one of the twenty most widespread dementia types.

Chapter 8: EARLY-ONSET ALZHEIMER'S DISEASE (EOAD)

If Alzheimer's disease (AD) is a demon, early-onset Alzheimer's disease (EOLD) is the devil.

In this chapter, we define EOLD, discuss how it differs from typical AD, its prevalence, and its causes.

How Prevalent is early-onset Alzheimer's (FAD)?

Many call early-onset Alzheimer's a rare form of Alzheimer's, but this dementia series views it as a significant dementia category. Representing a minimum of 5-10% of Alzheimer's disease (AD), early-onset familial Alzheimer's (FAD) adds up to a significant number of people.

5.5 million Americans are living with Alzheimer's disease, meaning 200,000 to 550,000 live with FAD.

Genetic or Sporadic EOAD

The medical profession categorizes early-onset Alzheimer's disease (EOAD), either familial (genetic) or sporadic. Most EOAD patients suffer the sporadic version.

Early-onset familial Alzheimer's disease (EOFAD)

Researchers link three genes to early-onset familial Alzheimer's disease (EOFAD).

- Presenilin 1 (PS1)
- Presenilin 2 (PS2)
- Amyloid precursor protein (APP)

Science links the above genes to chromosomes 1, 14, and 21, which we soon discuss.

The three genes are associated with only 1-3% of Alzheimer's cases but account for 60-70% of early-onset Alzheimer's disease (EOAD)[93].

Thus, when we discuss EOAD, we usually mean the familial variety.

Early-onset sporadic Alzheimer's disease

Sporadic means no genetic link. Accounting for most of typical Alzheimer's, but only 30-40% of early-onset Alzheimer's, the sporadic variety remains an uncompleted global-size puzzle with too many missing pieces.

While genes might still play a role in early-onset sporadic Alzheimer's, it is considered minor. In these cases, other factors such as toxins, oral infections, and elevated blood sugar are responsible.

Neurologist Dale Bredenson refers to these causes as 36 holes in the roof and argues you cannot repair a leaky roof by focusing on one hole. Rather than focus all energy on the amyloid plaque and tau tangles, Bredenson argues we must personalize a treatment plan for each patient.

By running tests to measure one's toxin exposure, blood sugar, and other contributors, and treating each, Bredenson argues we can prevent or reverse Alzheimer's, and by extension, a model to treat other dementias.

How does Early-onset Alzheimer's Disease (EOAD) differ from Typical Alzheimer's Disease (AD)?

The name suggests the most important difference. If we think of three generations of a family, Alzheimer's attacks the grandparent, and FAD the parent.

Symptoms do not show in most typical Alzheimer's patients until age 65 or older, but early-onset manifest symptoms in people 30-60 years old.

Early-onset strikes people in their prime, while fighting to the top of their profession, in the thick of raising children, and otherwise fully engaged in life.

Many psychologists and neurologists warn the shock is much greater when young people receive an early-onset Alzheimer's or another dementia diagnosis. Depression and anxiety often follow the first symptoms or diagnosis.

Age is an important difference between early-onset AD and typical AD but on one of several important differences.

Early-onset Alzheimer's also causes more myoclonus than typical AD. We discuss these sudden twitches more in the symptoms section.

There is also a much greater genetic connection to early-onset AD than typical AD.

What Causes Early-onset Familial Alzheimer's?

Whereas genetics plays a small role in typical Alzheimer's and most dementias, there is a strong link in early-onset Alzheimer's. Mutated genes in chromosomes 1, 14, and 21 cause early-onset Alzheimer's.

As with most dementia, protein deposits and tangles are front and center.

Chromosome 21 mutations most resemble typical Alzheimer's because of the resulting amyloid protein (APP) deposits. In contrast, mutated chromosome 1 causes presenilin 2, and chromosome 14 mutations cause presenilin 1 deposits.

Chromosome

Protective and snug in the nucleus, chromosomes carry DNA molecule and coils around histones (proteins) for support called nucleosomes[94].

Receiving one of each chromosome type from our mother and father, we are born with 46 chromosomes.

Chromosomes are either autosomes or allosomes. Autosomes are chromosomes 1-22, while allosomes include chromosomes X and Y.

Females carry two copies of chromosome X, while males have one chromosome X and one Y. Thus females carry chromosome XX and males XY.

Thousands of genes stretch from one end of a chromosome to the other, carrying necessary DNA instructions to construct the human body and vital proteins and other maintenance[95].

View the photo below to see where chromosome resides within the nucleus.

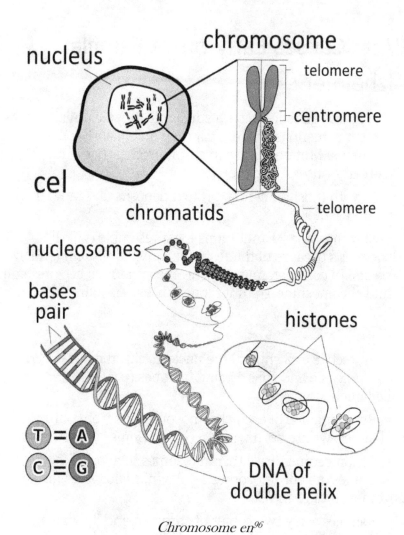

Chromosome en[96]

Let's discuss the three chromosomes linked to early-onset Alzheimer's disease (EOAD), chromosomes 1, 14, and 21.

Chromosome 1

Including 249 billion DNA base pairs, the largest chromosome, chromosome 1, represents eight percent of DNA cells. Chromosome 1 contains 2,000 to 2,100 total genes[97].

In regards to early-onset Alzheimer's disease (EOAD), we're interested in the PSEN2 gene.

(PSEN2) Gene

A protein-coding gene, PSEN2, delivers code to produce APH-1, PEN-2, nicastrin, and presenilin proteins. Presenilin is associated with EOAD.

Presenilin 2

A multiple gamma-secretase complex, presenilin 2 slices the amyloid precursor protein (APP) into smaller units called peptides[98]. Cleaving amyloid precursor protein (APP) prevents the accumulation associated with Alzheimer's.

Something occurs, causing presenilin 2 to malfunction, allowing Alzheimer's related protein accumulations.

Chromosome 14

Including 107 DNA building blocks, chromosome 14 represents up to 3.5 percent cellular DNA, a total o 800-900 genes. Each gene delivers instructions to produce important proteins.

The chromosome gene connected to Alzheimer's is PSENI.

PSENI Gene

The PSENI gene makes the Presenilin 1 protein, a proteolytic subunit of y-secretase.

Presenilin 1 Protein

Similar to what presenilin 2, presenilin 1 breaks amyloid precursor protein (APP) into smaller pieces, preventing the buildup associated with AD.

For reasons little or unknown, presenilin 1 sometimes turns mutant and stops doing its job. Unmolested, APP clumps together and leads to Alzheimer's.

Chromosome 21

The smallest human chromosome and autosome, totaling 1.5% of cellular DNA, chromosome 21 contains 48 million nucleotides. Also called trisomy 21, there are 225 total genes in chromosome 21, compared to thousands in the larger chromosomes[99].

Linked to Down syndrome, Trisomy 21 also plays a large role in 50% of Down syndrome survivors getting Alzheimer's if they live to forty.

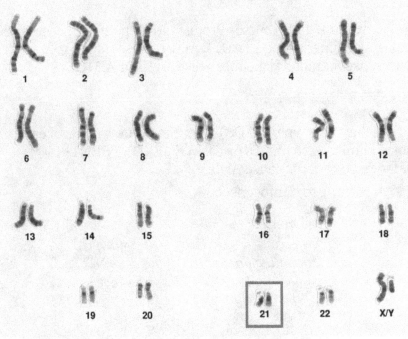

National Human Genome Research Institute[100]

Down syndrome with Alzheimer's disease is one of the 19 dementia types we cover in this series. Down syndrome represents one pathway to early-onset Alzheimer's disease (EOAD).

Early-onset Familial Alzheimer's Disease (EOFAD) Types

Early-onset familial Alzheimer's disease (EOFAD) is the genetic version and strikes people between ages thirty and sixty. Familial indicates Alzheimer's for more than one family member, usually a parent and child.

Authorities label Alzheimer's types 1, 3, and 4 as early-onset familial Alzheimer's disease (EOFAD).

Alzheimer's type 1 (AD1)

Amyloid Beta Precursor Protein (APP) pathogenic variants cause Alzheimer's type 1 (AD1). AD1 represents 10-15% of early-onset familial Alzheimer's disease (EOFAD) cases[101].

Alzheimer's type 3 (AD3)

Alzheimer's type 3 (AD3) accounts for up to 70% of early-onset familial Alzheimer's disease (EOFAD). PSEN1 pathogenic variants cause AD3.

According to Centogene[102]:

> Early-onset familial Alzheimer's disease-3 (AD3) is caused by heterozygous pathogenic variants in the presenilin-1 gene (PSEN1) on chromosome 14q24, and these pathogenic variants account for 30-70% of all early onsets AD cases 1, 4, 5. The protein encoded by PSEN1 acts as part of the gamma-secretase cleavage system for amyloid-β A4 protein. Clinical features of AD3 include {the} relatively rapid progression of memory and cognitive function loss associated with seizures, myoclonus, and language deficits 6. Several families have had associated spastic paraplegia with "cotton wool" amyloid plaques 7.

A progressive neurological disorder, AD3 produces "intraneuronal neurofibrillary tangles, extracellular amyloid plaques and vascular amyloid deposits," causing significant cognitive decline [103]."

Alzheimer's type 4 (AD4)

The last early-onset familial Alzheimer's disease (EOFAD) subtype is Alzheimer's type 4 (AD4). Whereas PSEN1 causes AD3, PSEN2 causes AD4, which accounts for 2% of Alzheimer's incidents.

PSEN2 causes plaque deposits and tangles, leading to brain damage causing Alzheimer's-related cognitive issues. We soon discuss PSEN1 and PSEN2 more in the early-onset Alzheimer's disease (EPAD) section.

We covered the EOFAD subtypes Alzheimer's types 1, 3, and 4 in this section. Next, let's examine late-onset familial Alzheimer's disease subtypes.

Non (EOAD) Genetic Causes

Researchers link toxins, high blood pressure, and oral infections to Alzheimer's (early and typical versions).

Noted neurologist and researcher Dale Bredesen identified 35 mechanisms leading to Alzheimer's. Bredesen likens the mechanisms to 35 holes in the roof. For Bredesen, defeating Alzheimer's is a matter of identifying the underlying causes and treating each problem.

Bredesen's approach reversed Alzheimer's in dozens of patients by addressing the 35 underlying causes. To my knowledge, this is the only program to reverse AD.

III. EOAD SYMPTOMS

Chapter 8: EARLY-ONSET ALZHEIMER'S DISEASE (EOAD) SYMPTOMS

The main difference between early-onset and typical Alzheimer's disease (EOAD) is the symptoms show before age 65 in the former. There are two types of early-onset Alzheimer's; common and genetics. Most cases are common.

EOAD Early Symptoms

In the early stage, one might forget newly learned information or dates. A person asks for the same information, again and again. They experience difficulty solving basic problems, such as keeping track of bills or following a favorite recipe

Somebody with EOAD loses track of the date or time of year. EOAD symptoms cause some to forget where they are or how they got there. Depth perception or other vision problems often occur in the early stages.

Somebody with EOAD struggles to join conversations or finding the right word. In the early stages, EOAD patients misplace things and cannot retrace steps to find the lost item.

EOAD patients suffer progressively poor judgment and changes in mood and personality. EOAD patients also suffer from mood swings and behavior issues. As a consequence, they withdraw from social and work situations.

Please read the symptoms and stages section for typical AD for more information about how the symptoms progress.

Chapter 9: EOAD SYMPTOMS

Let's discuss the more prevalent AD symptoms in greater detail.

Typical Alzheimer's Disease (AD) Symptoms

1. Delusions
2. Hallucinations
3. Memory Loss
4. Mood and Personality Changes
5. Poor Judgement
6. Losing things
7. Physical Abilities
8. Word Troubles
9. Time and Place issues
10. Visual Impairment

There are many warning signs you, or somebody close, need to pay attention to regarding Alzheimer's. Watch for dramatic changes to memory, habits, moods, and perceptions. If troubling patterns develop, act fast.

Alzheimer's disease symptoms manifest differently in each inflicted person. While the symptoms might show in a different order, most Alzheimer's patients develop the ten symptoms.

Delusions

People with Alzheimer's suffer delusions that make them tough to manage. They view the world with paranoid eyes and often believe falsehoods that hurt those attempting to care for them[104].

People living with Alzheimer's suffering such delusions accuse family and caretakers of stealing their possessions.

Or falsely accuse the next-door neighbor of trying to take their husband or wife.

Or believe you are not who you claim.

People with Alzheimer's latch on to paranoia and fear and lash out at others. Nothing you say, not even presenting evidence to prove them wrong, will change their minds. To others, the belief might be preposterous, but the Alzheimer's-related delusions are real to those suffering them.

Loved ones must remember Alzheimer's is a serious disease, and those suffering possess little or no control over the symptoms. You cannot engage in arguments or otherwise chastise them for actions beyond their control.

The disease kills them in slow, methodical steps by robbing their ability to think, reason, perceive, and otherwise exercise the cognitive skills necessary for consistent normal-thinking. Alzheimer's patients accuse their loved ones and caregivers of awful things, but it's not their fault.

Please remember a demon called Alzheimer's attacked, and it is the disease driving the erratic and cruel behavior, not the person you've always known.

A point I shall risk repetition in this book: **Do not blame Alzheimer's patients for their behavior!**

Paranoia

One form of delusion, someone suffering paranoia associated with Alzheimer's, might believe others are out to get them. They suspect others of lying, cheating, cruelty, stealing, and other high crimes and misdemeanors.

They might look in the mirror and see a police car that is not there.

Or insist somebody is living in the attic.

11 things you should do or not do when a loved one suffers delusions and paranoia:

1. Ask the doctor if medications could cause the symptoms.
2. Check for cause and try to ease their concerns.
3. Establish regular routines
4. Feed them well-balanced meals. Lots of berries, nuts, vegetables, and wild-caught fish.
5. Keep answers short and elementary.
6. Reassure them.
7. Steer attention to something more positive.
8. Verify they are suffering a delusion, and not something real.
9. Do not argue.
10. Do not convince.
11. Do not take offense.

The days of winning philosophical and other battles with the afflicted person are over! Do not argue, convince, or take offense at the delusional behavior.

Try to remember as offensive and hurtful as it might be to you; what they experience is a thousand times more frightening. Cognitive abilities decline, and now they see unreal things that are their new reality. These unreal things they experience are as real to them as they might be ridiculous to others.

When they believe somebody is living in the attic, or

somebody is not who they claim to be, no matter how false, it could not be more real to those experiencing the delusions.

If they accuse you of being an imposter, it matters not if they have known you their entire life.

Be prepared! Once Alzheimer's strikes the sweetest person in the world, their meanest, most unreasonable moments test the most patient of souls and puncture those with the thickest skin.

Doctors treat symptoms with medication, which minimizes certain behavioral disorders. Some drugs are a godsend, while others only make the situation worse and risk too many dangerous side effects.

While people often confuse delusions and hallucinations, there are important differences, which we now examine.

Alzheimer's Hallucinations

Hallucinations differ from delusions.

Whereas delusions cause believed falsehoods, people with Alzheimer's-related hallucinations experience sensory emotions that seem real to them. Alzheimer's patients not only see unreal people or things but smells odors, hears noises, holds conversations, taste, and feel to round out the hallucination[105].

Most of the hallucinations involve seeing and hearing people and things not there, although they might think they smell something they associate with evil or their childhood.

Hallucinations do not include mistaking something for something else, but believing something is there when it is not. In their heads, the imaginary things they see, touch, hear, smell, and taste are as real as their non-hallucinations.

What causes the hallucinations?

- Dim or flickering lighting could cause hallucinations in people with Alzheimer's.
- Broken routines, such as unfamiliar people and places, could explain the problem.
- Medication is a strong possibility, so report the issue and ask the doctor if medications could be the issue.
- Sundowning: a condition where those with Alzheimer's symptoms worsen later in the day.

The reasons for the hallucinations will differ for each person, but try the recommendations above and go from there.

The triggers differ for each person.

I suggest you keep a journal and make notes about each episode. Where did it take place? Who was present before and at the time of hallucination? List as much detail as possible. While it might not set off immediate alarms by itself, it might make more sense when you or the doctor reviews the journal.

The journal also can be therapeutic for loved ones and

caregivers. Keeping a journal benefits the person with Alzheimer's and helps loved ones and caregivers focus on important matters.

Do NOT use this journal to probe your emotional stress. Instead, use a personal diary or therapy to address your turmoil. Make the journal about the patient.

List as much as possible, including their eating and sleeping patterns, response to medication and therapy, delusion and hallucination triggers, physical mobility and balance, cognitive strengths and weaknesses, and anything you think important.

What should you do when a loved one is suffering Alzheimer's-related hallucinations?

It is the same list as suggested for handling delusions:

- Ask the doctor if medications could cause the symptoms.
- Check for cause and try to ease their concerns.
- Do not argue.
- Do not convince.
- Check for cause and try to ease their concerns.
- Do not take offense.
- Establish regular routines
- Feed them well-balanced meals. Lots of nuts, berries, vegetables, and wild-caught fish.
- Keep answers short and elementary.
- Reassure them.
- Steer attention to something more positive.

Verify they are suffering a delusion, and not something real.

Losing Things

We're not referring to misplacing keys or something minor that most do from time to time, but losing things and not having a clue how. If somebody exhibits such symptoms, see a doctor[106].

The inability to retrace one's steps when they lose something is one of ten Alzheimer's symptoms that should ring the alarms. People with Alzheimer's often lose something, find themselves incapable of re-tracking their steps, and accuse somebody of stealing the missing item.

How does one know if it is normal aging issues or Alzheimer's?

The Cleveland Clinic explained what is considered normal memory issues, and something more serious like Alzheimer's[107]:

What's typical: Misplacing things from time to time, such as a pair of glasses or the remote control.

When to seek help: Putting things in unusual places, losing things, and being unable to go back over one's steps to find them again, accusing others of stealing.

Like other Alzheimer's symptoms in this book, one must remember it is the disease, not the person. No matter what kind of person they were before Alzheimer's, the disease takes over and removes the ability to process thought and regulate behavior.

Somebody with Alzheimer's might hide clothing in the freezer, the remote control in the dryer, keys in the oven, or any other imaginable misplacement.

By this point, a person should have already seen a doctor.

Once a doctor diagnoses Alzheimer's, it is important for caregivers and loved ones to lock up valuables, and lock away or remove toxins, and to minimize the number of places to hide things.

According to the National Institute on Aging, "there might be a logical reason for this behavior. For instance, the person may look for something specific, although he or she may not be able to tell you what it is[108]," causing difficulty for those suffering Alzheimer's and loved ones.

Let's next look at perhaps the most immediate and prominent Alzheimer's symptom.

Memory Loss

My shining days may be dimming, for sure, but life for me is not done/May God grant me peace, whatever those sunset days may bring.

— From a poem written by Alzheimer's patient John MacInnes

A retired executive and former pastor, MacInnes recognized he had a problem when he planned out a spectacular presentation as he had done numerous times on powerpoint. But, the presentation did not go as dozens of others had before. "In mid-sentence, I had problems," McInnes said, "I had a well-rehearsed script in front of me, but I couldn't get the words right, couldn't get them out. That kind of shook me up[109]."

From there, John struggled to multi-task, one of his former strengths. Next, he becomes disoriented while driving a few times. Age 80, John made an appointment, and his doctor diagnosed him with Alzheimer's. The early diagnosis allowed him to treat his symptoms and plan for the road ahead.

But, how do we know it is not normal memory problems?

We all forget things. At our worst, we might even worry about ourselves. But it becomes more problematic if we can't remember recent events, names of people we know well, important dates we once processed, and need to make notes to remember the most basic information[110].

Undiagnosed and unsuspected, in the early stages, amyloid plaque and neurofibrillary tangles are doing progressive damage to brain cells (neurons or nerve cells)[111].

Memory of Smell

Losing the sense of smell is an early Alzheimer's memory symptom.

John Holger, MD, led a University Hospital Hamburg-Eppendorf review of 81 studies on Alzheimer's effect on the memory of smell.

Holger explained that Alzheimer's originates in the entorhinal cortex, the part of the brain that processes and communicates smell.

The meta-analysis of 81 studies confirmed people with Alzheimer's are "impaired on odor identification and recognition tasks," Holger said. "The impairment of smell recognition is of clinical importance, as patients often report malodorous sensations and changes in, e.g., the taste of foods leading to behavioral alterations. Consequences may range from increasing malnutrition to the development of delusions of poisoning that may trigger aggressive behavior[112]."

It is easy for loved ones to mistake the sudden changes in food tastes to somebody becoming difficult. They might one day turn hostile towards what had been their favorite meal.

"This feature of the neural network of smell memory," Holger said, "reflects the evolutionary pressure towards the secure recognition of 'bad' smells pointing to poisonous or rotten food that is pivotal for the survival of the organism."

Other Memory Loss Symptoms

Memory loss is one of the first symptoms of Alzheimer's. We already covered the memory of smell, and now will examine other examples of memory loss caused by Alzheimer's[113,114,115,116]:

- Can no longer manage medication
- Does not recognize familiar surroundings and gets lost while walking, driving, or shopping
- Does not remember anniversaries and birthdays
- Forgets recent events
- Forgets recent conversations
- Hides possessions such as keys or wallet in strange places such as the garage and forgetting
- Misses appointments
- Moodier than usual
- Repeats questions
- Struggles with normal tasks such as cooking or making coffee
- Word problems such as calling a cat a dog

Whatever one's normal memory before, it deteriorates once Alzheimer's symptoms show. If you or a loved one experiences any of the above or similar symptoms, see a competent doctor at once.

Whatever is causing the problem is serious, a diagnosis is important whether the problem is Alzheimer's or something else.

We next examine mood and personality changes somebody with Alzheimer's experiences.

Mood And Personality Changes

People with Alzheimer's struggle with moods and their personality changes. They're suspicious, anxious, often fearful, depressed, perplexed, insecure, and off-balance[117].

The aggression comes in two types:

Verbal Aggression

People with Alzheimer's struggle to process thoughts and lose their ability to screen what they say. Like a child, if something pops in their mind, they say it without considering its appropriateness.

An agreeable person who never said an unkind word to anybody might become belligerent, contrary, insulting, arrogant, or otherwise aggressive. Somebody who once shied from confrontation might instigate conflict.

Physical Aggression

The most gentle person in the world might go into a rage and destroy property or even threaten others. For some, they can no more control their physical aggression than screen what they say.

5 to 10 percent of those with Alzheimer's turn violent.

Michael Cohen described to CNN how his father went from a peaceful man to somebody his mother had to call 911 for breaking glass and threatening behavior. "It's like the 'Invasion of the Body Snatchers,'" said Cohen. "It looks like Dad, sounds like Dad, but it's not Dad[118]."

See your doctor and circle the family if you see signs in a loved one of violence. When somebody with Alzheimer's become aggressive, search for the cause and help defuse the situation.

Before we go to the next section, let's review the list of mood and personality changes associated with Alzheimer's.

List of Mood Changes Caused by Alzheimer's

Mood changes related to Alzheimer's[119][120]:

- Aggression, anger, agitation
- Anxiety
- Calm and then upset without reason
- Delusions
- Emotionally unstable
- Fatigued all the time
- Hallucinations
- Happy, then sad for no reason
- More anxious than usual
- Physical outbursts
- Sleep issues
- Unprovoked anger and mood swings
- Unusual pacing

Let's examine each symptom.
Aggression, Anger, & Agitation

Stress often causes aggression, agitation, and anger. When a loved one with Alzheimer's experiences these symptoms, instead of getting upset, you must recognize the cause.

According to the Alzheimer's Society, "Aggressive behavior might be a person's way of trying to achieve what they need."

Whatever their needs, they cannot accomplish it on their own or communicate it to others.

Possible causes

They might experience[121][122]:

- Boredom
- Constipation
- Depression
- Distrust of health care professionals
- Loneliness
- Loss of inhibitions
- Hallucinations
- Reaction to being treated like they are helpless
- Side effects of medication
- Thirst
- Unfamiliar setting

Many real and unreal things could turn their world upside down and torment their emotions. Figure out the cause and calm them by addressing the problem, if possible.

Only 5-10 percent of people carrying Alzheimer's will become violent but be prepared.

Safety

When somebody living with Alzheimer's exhibits aggressive behavior, the National Institute on Aging recommends: "Protect yourself and others. If you have to stay at a safe distance from the person until the behavior stops. Also, try to protect the person from hurting himself or herself[123]."

The NIH warning is spot-on but also shows the complexity as they both encourage caregivers to keep a safe distance when an AD patient turns violent but reminds the important protection role.

Find a balance between protecting yourself and the AD patient, as circumstances can turn your duty and common sense into direct conflict. If necessary, keep a safe distance, but try to figure out the source of their agitation and do your best to calm them.

If you feel threatened, speak to the family and medical officials. Doctors must treat 5-10% of AD patients who turn violent different than regular AD patients, most likely through behavior medication. While the typical AD patient should avoid the drugs in question, doctors must consider them to minimize violent outbursts endangering both patients and caregivers.

Anxiety

Somewhat related to aggression, anger, and agitation is anxiety. We did not include anxiety in that grouping because it often has different causes.

Several studies link anxiety to Alzheimer's, including the Pittsburg study released in the *American Journal of Psychiatry*. The Pittsburg study followed seniors in Pittsburg to determine if anxiety raises the level of the protein amyloid-beta.

Dr. Nancy Donovan, the lead author, explained[124]:

> *Higher amyloid beta burden was associated with increasing anxious-depressive symptoms over time in cognitively normal older individuals. Prior depression history was related to higher but not worsening symptom ratings. These results suggest a direct or indirect association of elevated amyloid beta levels with worsening anxious-depressive symptoms and support the hypothesis that emerging*

> *neuropsychiatric symptoms represent an early manifestation of preclinical Alzheimer's disease.*

Scientists believe anxiety increases the amount of amyloid beta protein disrupting neurons and is one of two primary features of Alzheimer's.

Those suffering anxiety related to Alzheimer's might suffer "generalized anxiety disorder, panic disorder, social anxiety disorder, and specific fears or phobias[125]."

Calm and then upset without reason

Without provocation, somebody with Alzheimer's can go from absolute calm to howling at the moon.

Delusions

In part because of the disease, and also because of side effects to drugs, Alzheimer's causes delusions.

For more information on the relationship of delusions, refer to the chapter covering how it is symptomatic of Alzheimer's.

Emotionally unstable

We all experience difficulty controlling our emotions, but those with Alzheimer's become unstable, and their condition worsens as the disease progresses.

Fatigued all the time

Somebody with Alzheimer's might not sleep well at night, but want to sleep during the day. While they suffer many hallucinations, being fatigued is real. They are not getting enough sleep for the brain to filter out the toxins and reboot. We all require 7-8 hours of sleep to practice sound physical and mental health.

Hallucinations

Somebody with Alzheimer's suffering hallucinations will

see, smell, and feel things that do not exist.

Refer to the Hallucinations section for more information.

Happy, then sad for no reason

As with other emotional extremes, for no logical reason, Alzheimer's patients often go from happy to sad in the time to snap one's finger.

More anxious than usual

People with Alzheimer's often find it impossible to relax, as they remain on edge, uncomfortable, and impatient.

Physical outbursts

As already described, Alzheimer's patients lose restraint and can become dangerous to property, themselves, and those around them.

Sleep issues

Alzheimer's causes sleep problems, making it impossible to sleep at night.

Unusual pacing

Before they lose the ability, many with Alzheimer's pace back and forth and otherwise cannot keep still.

Now we've covered mood and personality changes caused by Alzheimer's. Let's move to the next symptom, poor judgment.

Poor Judgment

Impaired judgment, a cornerstone of Alzheimer's, often shows before memory loss.

In a study released in the *PubMed* analyzed data from 1990 to 2011. They found: "Loss of judgment capacity is common in

EARLY-ONSET ALZHEIMER'S DISEASE (EOAD)

dementia {Alzheimer's} when cognitive functions allowing the use of purposeful behaviors progressively fail."

The poor judgment manifests in different ways but is noticeable because they are out-of-character. In areas where somebody has a history of sound decision-making, they slip.

If a person who always pays bills on time becomes incapable, this is a possible indicator of Alzheimer's. Associated poor judgment might include poor hygiene and basic decline. A tidy person might dress sloppy and allow their surroundings to become cluttered or even unsanitary[126].

Somebody with Alzheimer's judgment becomes reckless, improper, or indecent.

Somebody suffering Alzheimer's might:

- Allow personal hygiene to slip
- Allow cons or salespeople to take advantage of them
- Believe the utility people want to rob him/her
- Believe a bill they've paid for years is not theirs
- Difficulty making a grocery list
- Dress inappropriately (go to a mall in pajamas or wear a winter jacket in the sweltering heat of summer)
- Go from a good cook to horrible because they stop using recipes
- Insist the neighbor is stealing their newspaper (not delivered in a decade)
- Make questionable financial decisions
- Place themselves in danger by climbing in a car with a stranger
- Struggle with planning

When considering the chances of Alzheimer's, look for uncharacteristic odd behavior.

Once diagnosed, expect your loved one's behavior impairment to worsen as the disease advances.

Physical Abilities

Some physical warning signs are sudden mobility or coordination problems. Examples include the inability to make the bed, fold laundry, shower, dress, and conduct other simple tasks you or your loved one have been doing with ease[127]. They might perform these tasks but won't do them right, not as they've always done before.

Physical problems caused by Alzheimer's

A few Alzheimer's physical difficulties[128][129][130]:

- Balance problems
- Bladder control issues
- Bowel problems
- Coordination issues
- Stiff muscles
- Drags feet while walking
- Seizures
- Trouble sitting
- Trouble standing
- Unmanaged twitching

Alzheimer's patients develop these at different intervals. The earlier diagnosed for Alzheimer's, the better chance doctors have for treating the symptoms. While not a cure, treatments exist to reduce the severity of some symptoms.

As the disease progresses, people with Alzheimer's suffer six particular physical threats[131][132].

1. Bedsores
2. Dehydration
3. Infections because the immune system fails
4. Injuries from frequent falls.
5. Malnutrition
6. Pneumonia

Next, let's examine word troubles people with Alzheimer's experience.

Time And Place Issues

Another Alzheimer's symptom is confusion over where one is or how they got there. They struggle to grasp anything or concept that isn't in front of them[133].

Time and place confusion terrifies. Not knowing where one is or how you got there, bewilders, and disorients Alzheimer's patients.

They remember who they are, and most memory remains intact the first time or two the Alzheimer's patient gets lost.

It also is dangerous.

When we become lost under these symptoms, we depend on strangers to figure out how to get us home or call somebody we know.

The right stranger is a godsend, while the wrong one poses a monetary or physical threat.

Often, time and place issues are what sparks the visit to the doctor's office. If the person suffering the symptoms does not go on their own, a loved one steps in and says, "This is serious. You must see the doctor."

Visual Impairment

Watch out for the sudden inability to process color, contrast, and distance. Driving becomes difficult (dangerous) in the early stages. Finding one's way to the bathroom in their home is a more advanced symptom. If you, or somebody close to you, struggle to grasp the full concept of visual images and distance becomes impaired, please see your physician immediately[134].

Visual impairment increases the risk of and intensity of Alzheimer's[135].

When the eyes and brain do not work together, one experiences "difficulties with vision and perception, which causes them to misinterpret the world[136]."

Scientists believe this vision impairment causes some hallucinations associated with Alzheimer's.

Even with healthy eyes, people with Alzheimer's can suffer the same visual impairment. As the University of California Memory and Aging Center explained: "The shrinking brain can no longer interpret and process the information received from the person's healthy eyes[137]."

The medical term for this visual impairment is Posterior Cortical Atrophy (PCA).

Posterior Cortical Atrophy (PCA)

What is PCA?

The *Journal of the Alzheimer's Association* describes PCA: [138]

> *Posterior Cortical Atrophy (PCA) is a rare neurodegenerative disease associated with Alzheimer's disease pathology that presents with progressive deterioration in visual perception. Patients with PCA present with complex visual impairments such as Balint syndrome, Gerstmann syndrome, simultanagnosia, neglect, and topographical disorientation.*

Below are the most common Alzheimer's-related PCA symptoms[139][140][141][142].

- Cannot perceive three-dimension objects
- Cannot recognize objects
- Bumps into things
- Cannot recognize people
- Confuse a shadow for a hole in the floor
- Cannot articulate what they see
- Confuse a reflection for a stranger
- Depth perception breaks down (struggles with concepts like distance)
- Trouble detecting movement

- Lose the ability to detect colors
- Bright lights cause problems
- Sight field depth shrinks
- Difficulty reaching for objects
- Failure to detect contrasts
- Trouble sitting

Posterior Cortical Atrophy makes Alzheimer's even more difficult and challenging. Everything we take for granted concerning vision breaks down because Alzheimer's destroys neurons serving as the communication network between the brain and eyes.

If a loved one with Alzheimer's suffers Posterior Cortical Atrophy, ask their doctor for a full list of symptoms and things such as bright objects known to disturb them.

We've covered Alzheimer's-related vision impairment, so let's turn our attention to word troubles.

Word Troubles

If somebody starts repeating themselves, forgetting words, calling objects by their wrong name, and otherwise experiencing regular vocabulary issues, get them checked for Alzheimer's[143].

One thing might get locked in their head, and their mind loops back around to the dominating topic. Every few minutes, or thirty seconds, they might tell you the same thing and in their mind be telling it the first time.

In my mother's case, her mind locked on to my father, who died while she was well into stage three Alzheimer's. She repeated the same story: "J.C. (her brother) introduced me to Lawrence (my father and her husband). "

Each time she spoke with great conviction and thought it was the first time to speak the thought, sometimes a couple of times per minute. Watching her saddened the rest of the family and me, but nothing like in later stages when she no longer could articulate even this one dear thought.

When repeating the phrase, she sounded like the mom we always knew, but only while uttering the same words, and if we overlooked, she had already said it dozens of times.

The other thing she repeated during this period following my father's death: "I'm just hanging in there for my boys."

Mom demonstrated a person in stage 3 or 4 Alzheimer's still has deep thoughts and feelings, but in a loop, they cannot escape.

Parts of the brain unaffected allow a person to hold on to regular thoughts and actions, but the damaged areas break down their ability to perform what before were the simplest of tasks.

Let's review word problems associated with Alzheimer's

The shortlist[144]:

- Can no longer grasp simple words
- Can no longer write checks
- Cannot calculate (tips and budgets become impossible)
- Deteriorating mathematical skills
- Cannot name familiar objects
- Forgets people's names they've known for decades
- Cannot follow conversations
- Difficulty reading
- Mispronounced or mumbled words
- Mistake words (bedroom for bathroom, chair for lamp)
- Repeat the same question or statement dozens of times
- Speech becomes slower
- Spelling worsens

- Word use shrinks
- Words in the wrong order
- Talk less
- "Talking around a word (e.g., 'We went to the place where you can get bread' for the words 'grocery store')"

When words become difficult, communication breaks down, and the person becomes frustrated. Even when they know what to say, they struggle to say what they mean, and their ability to articulate goes into a steady decline.

Chapter 10: EOAD STAGES

Having covered symptoms, in this section, we demonstrate how the symptoms progress through the different Alzheimer's stages.

The model in this section works for typical Alzheimer's, early-onset Alzheimer's, and Down syndrome with Alzheimer's. All three share similar symptoms and progression. The primary difference is when the symptoms strike, as early-onset AD and Down syndrome AD strike people younger than typical AD.

The one part in this chapter that does not apply to early-onset AD and Down syndrome with AD are the fictional characters (based on real characters) who are dealing with typical AD. Otherwise, the information applies to all three.

According to Johns Hopkins Medical and other authorities, there are four primary stages[145]:

- Preclinical Alzheimer's
- Early-Stage Alzheimer's
- Middle-Stage Alzheimer's
- Late-Stage Alzheimer's

Others use a seven-stage model. Weaving the different models together, we use a three-stage model with seven substages.

3 Stages, 7 Substages Alzheimer's Model

Besides the four primary stages, there are seven substages.

Alzheimer's Substages

1. Substage One: No cognitive decline.
2. Substage Two: Very mild cognitive decline.
3. Substage Three: Mild cognitive decline.

Early-Stage Alzheimer's
   4. Substage Four: Moderate cognitive decline.

Middle-Stage Alzheimer's
   5. Substage Five: Moderate/severe cognitive decline.
   6. Substage Six: Severe cognitive decline.

Late-Stage Alzheimer's
   7. Substage Seven: Severest cognitive decline.

Each stage and substage marks greater advancement and severity in Alzheimer's. The damage to the neurons is destroying the brain's ability to communicate with other parts of the brain, the body, and the organs.

This section focuses on Alzheimer's four primary stages and seven sub-stages.

Let's begin with preclinical Alzheimer's.

Alzheimer's Stage 1

Stage one includes substages one through three.

Substage 1: Preclinical Alzheimer's

The earliest doctors diagnose Alzheimer's is stage four. The medical community considers the first three substages preclinical Alzheimer's.

Not having a blood or urine test for Alzheimer's like most diseases makes neurologists a day late and a dollar short in diagnosing dementia, although at least one test shows promise in studies. How soon a test works its way to the market depends on how fast larger human studies are funded and conducted and how long it takes for FDA approval. However, the process could take years!

The test must distinguish between typical Alzheimer's, hippocampal sparing Alzheimer's, limbic-predominant age-related TDP-43 (LATE), and posterior cortical atrophy. We also need a blood or urine test for the other fourteen primary dementias.

Until we can definitively diagnose Alzheimer's and the other dementias in stage one, a cure for each will remain out of science's reach.

During this stage, amyloid plaque is forming outside the brain's neurons, and another form of protein is clumping from the inside.

While no symptoms will appear for some time, at least none that does not resemble normal aging or emotional stress, the prelude to Alzheimer's is brewing in the brain.

By the time symptoms show, the protein build-up has already damaged the brain neurons. The plaque is destroying the neurons' ability to serve as the giant communication network allowing different parts of the brain to communicate with each other and to internal organs and body parts. Until we find a cure, from the time Alzheimer's manifests, it is a slow march to the grave.

It is vital to stop Alzheimer's in its tracks, preventing protein plaques and lumps to damage the neurons. The priority to cure or block Alzheimer's while the brain still has near 100 percent cognitive abilities.

Waiting until the rogue protein deposits form and symptoms show is unacceptable. The governments, corporations, and wealthy individuals must invest in two things we do not yet have in the fight against Alzheimer's:

- A cheap, accurate test
- A cure

Need More Funding for Research

An affordable and accurate means of testing and a cure for Alzheimer's disease (AD) before damage should be top priorities for every nation. AD is a horrific disease that takes a person's mind, and then their motor skills put them through hell and kill them. This disease strikes an American every 68 seconds and somebody worldwide every 3 seconds.

What governments, nonpharmaceutical corporations, and wealthy people contribute towards research to find a test and cure for a disease that kills one out of every three seniors[146] is unacceptable. Fighting AD is war, and those who possess most of the world's wealth are not supporting the research to discover accurate testing before the disease manifests and a cure.

Americans and citizens of the world must demand better from our governments. Until then, 5.7 million Americans[147] and 50 million people worldwide[148] will suffer Alzheimer's stages outlined in the following chapters.

We hope one day soon, Alzheimer's is all but wiped out like the medical community once accomplished with the polio vaccine. A test for early diagnosis and a cure will prevent the stages we are about to explore.

Let's review the first three substages of Preclinical Alzheimer's.

Alzheimer's Substage 1

No Cognitive Decline

During this stage, Alzheimer's is the true silent killer, building up the plaque and tangles in the brain, undetected, creating the foundation for the disease to attack.

Victims remain unaware they have the disease in substage one, as symptoms do not yet appear, the disease goes undetected.

Alzheimer's might damage the brain for decades before symptoms show. It is during this period when we need to detect, treat, and cure Alzheimer's.

Any future cure will involve treating Alzheimer's in the early stages before the damage becomes too severe, for science might never provide a cure for late-stage Alzheimer's. Once AD destroys the brain, not even the best science of the future will be able to rebuild such a complicated and original organ.

Doug Brown, former Chief Policy and Research Officer of the Alzheimer's Society, discussed this point.

"Cure will not be a silver bullet," said Brown. "A cure for us is either something that can prevent someone from developing dementia in the first place, or can stop dementia in its tracks before it has caused too much damage[149]."

Brown suggested the answer for those with advanced Alzheimer's will be a variety of drugs and treatment but agreed the solution is in preventing the disease before it becomes irreversible brain damage.

One's cognitive health appears in good shape during substage one. Let's turn our attention to substage two.

Alzheimer's Substage Two

Very Mild Cognitive Decline

Let's see what happens during substage two.

Alzheimer's Substage Two Symptoms

- Forget names
- Forget familiar words
- Hide money and forget where
- Misplace keys
- Miss an appointment

During stage two, one might forget an appointment, where they place their keys, hide their money, and other minor things that many non-Alzheimer's seniors face age 65 and beyond.

The cognitive issues experienced during substage two are not severe enough to raise any major alarms. The person experiencing the symptoms and people around them view such minor cognitive issues as normal.

Nor would a doctor observe anything alarming during substage two. Without cheaper, more accurate testing, no symptoms show at this point that would prompt a doctor to order an expensive round of imaging tests.

Science has not yet advanced far enough for doctors to diagnose Alzheimer's during substages one through three.

Alzheimer's Substage Three

Substage three is when denial runs head-on into reality.

Mild Cognitive Decline

A person shows more symptoms during this stage, and the conditions worsen.

Substage three, the person carrying Alzheimer's and closest loved ones grow more concerned. Normal cognitive hiccups during substage two evolve into more problematic episodes.

Substage Three Symptoms

- Declining planning skills
- Declining organizing skills
- Losing valuables
- Trouble forming coherent sentences
- Trouble remembering names

During this stage, holding a complex job and socializing becomes difficult. Planning skills deteriorate.

When a loved one exhibits the above symptoms, it is time to see a doctor. While the doctor will not diagnose Alzheimer's at this stage, she or he can document and treat the symptoms.

Since everybody experiences mild cognitive issues when depressed, stressed, or suffering from various illnesses, we too often dismiss early Alzheimer's symptoms as nothing serious. This thinking can backfire and become the worst decision in one's life.

Several medical conditions share the symptoms, so we do not yet know enough to confirm Alzheimer's. If the problem is Alzheimer's, it has laid perhaps decades of groundwork and is prepared to destruct one person's life and turn their loved ones' lives upside down.

This section completes the three substages of preclinical Alzheimer's stage one. Let's move to what is considered Alzheimer's.

STAGE 2: EARLY-STAGE ALZHEIMER'S

Now, we reach the earliest point doctors can diagnose Alzheimer's. Previous symptoms that people attribute to normal aging become more pronounced and difficult to explain.

A person suffering the symptoms must see a doctor, and crucial they make an "early" diagnosis.

While science offers no cure at the moment, earlier the doctor diagnoses the disease, the earlier he or she can treat the symptoms, minimize their severity, and stall the disease.

The quantity of quality life left depends on how fast the person exhibiting symptoms sees a doctor, how fast the doctor diagnoses the disease, and what treatment they implement.

Alzheimer's Substage Four

Whereas the first three substages rock the boat, distorting reality, substage four ends life as we know it, sucking us into a journey we never want.

Moderate Cognitive Decline

Through substage three, a person develops cognitive issues, but doctors do not consider it Alzheimer's until substage four. Now is when a person finds normal activities difficult, such as balancing checkbooks and focusing.

The reason doctors cannot diagnose Alzheimer's before substage 4 is there is no definitive test (a recurring theme).

Let's review some Alzheimer's substage four's symptoms.

Alzheimer's Substage 4 Symptoms

- Asks for help when ordering food
- Cannot perform simple arithmetic
- Depression
- Deteriorating awareness and concern for current or recent events
- Difficulty balancing a checkbook and dealing with personal finances
- Struggles to plan long term
- Forget conversation or event from earlier
- Mood swings
- Trouble managing the bills
- Short-term memory problems (Might not remember somebody visited earlier, or what they had for breakfast)
- Trouble reciting life history
- Unable to count backward from 100 by sevens
- Unable to shop for groceries
- Withdrawn

Sources: Medical News Today[150], Alzheimer's Net[151], Aging Care[152], Medicine Net[153]

During this stage, a person still maintains most of their memory, communication, and motor skills, but the areas where they are slipping are pronounced and alarming.

It is crucial the person and their loved ones accept there is a problem, potentially fatal.

Denial is one of the worst enemies for somebody with substage four Alzheimer's. And loved ones must often say things that hurt, anger, or frightens the person suffering the symptoms.

If you are in this position as a loved one, be diplomatic but adamant that the person exhibiting symptoms see a doctor this, not next week. The important thing is to get them to the doctor without destroying your relationship.

It is difficult enough to admit mental problems, but almost impossible for some of us to admit to others.

Pride and denial work hand-in-hand too often in humans but stand in the way of perhaps the most important diagnosis of one's life.

Besides the person with Alzheimer's needing time to prepare before the disease gets too serious, family and friends need time to figure out how they will handle what will grow into 24/7 caretaking, as the loved one becomes as helpless as a newborn baby.

If somebody visits a doctor when in substage two or three, the medical officials know the cognitive issues and can diagnose Alzheimer's early in substage 4.

The earlier the detection, the better. Anybody facing Alzheimer's must give the medical professionals every chance to stall the disease and extend the amount of quality time left.

If neurologists diagnose a loved one with substage four Alzheimer's, cherish this stage. Now is the closest the inflicted person will ever be to what they once were. They still maintain most of their personality and what makes them unique.

One of the saddest things anybody ever has to do is watch a loved one disappear a little at a time.

Substage 4 Duration

Since substage four is the official starting point for Alzheimer's, we start the timetable here. The meantime for stage two and substage four is **two years.**

AD Stage 3

Middle-Stage Alzheimer's

The loved one takes another turn for the worse during stage three. Now is the last best chance to experience and enjoy any of the person's personality.

There are two substages in stage three, substages five and six.

AD Substage Five

Moderately Severe Cognitive Decline

Whereas one fights in substage four to maintain as much independence as possible, one grows progressively more dependent in substage five.

Stage 5 Symptoms

- Can no longer cook, even assisted
- Continuous confusion
- Develops hygiene problems (not flushing toilet, brushing teeth, etc.)
- Inappropriate dressing
- Trouble processing time and place
- Trouble remembering their anniversary, birthday, high school, college, and other personal histories
- Unable to dress themselves
- Unable to remember a phone number, address, and simple details

Substage 5 Duration

Substage five lasts a mean of 1.5 years.

Let's now turn our attention to substage six.

Substage Six

As challenging as prior substages posed, substage six demoralizes the soul.

Patient and caregivers struggle through each day, as the symptoms worsen. Bladder and bowel impairment grows severe enough to cause embarrassing accidents.

Wandering becomes a greater problem, so they require 24/7 care. Hallucinations and confusion render many moments impossible.

Severe Cognitive Decline

During this stage, recollecting names becomes difficult, even when a person recognizes somebody. They also struggle to remember where the steps, bathroom, and other places are, even when feet away.

Mistaking a brother for one's father, or wife for their mother, and otherwise confusing one's relationship is common.

Stage six is the last to communicate with your loved one as they still have moments where they recognize people and can hold semi-normal conversations.

During this period, the roles of parents and children often reverse. It is important for healthy spouses, children, and other loved ones to reassure them, let them know you loved them, read to them, play calming music, take them for walks, go through their favorite photo albums and try to stir warm memories.

They will find it difficult to go to the bathroom and suffer immeasurable shame, so tell them it is okay. If you're a sibling, remind them they once did the same for you.

A person who retired as a teacher or doctor twenty years earlier might wake up and believe they must head to the school or office.

The mental deterioration throughout stage six, while not as cruel as the final stage, demands constant supervision.

They are incapable of choosing what clothes to wear, what to eat, or much of anything.

They can, however, still sit, walk, and hold infrequent coherent thoughts. Enjoy this, for they will lose what's left in the next and final stage.

Substage Six Alzheimer's Symptoms

- Behavior issues[154]
- Cannot remember recent events
- Confusion
- Continued memory decline
- Loss of bladder control
- Loss of bowel control
- Need help with daily living (bathing, toiletry, feeding) [155]
- Repetitious (repeats the same phrase or physical motion like snapping fingers or flipping one's hand dismissively) [156]
- Significant personality changes
- Sundowning (symptoms worsen in late afternoon and evening) [157]
- Suspicious
- Trouble using the bathroom by themselves
- Trouble with surroundings[158]
- Unable to recognize friends and family
- Unable to remember personal details
- Wandering[159]

Substage 6 Duration

The mean duration for substage six is 2.5 years.

Alzheimer's Stage 4

Literature refers to the last act, or perhaps the climax. Everything snowballs towards the ending at this point. What we hope has been a productive, happy life winds down.

The only question at this point is the cause of death. While Alzheimer's is the root-cause, people often die from a symptom such as pneumonia, which the authorities will list as the cause on the death certificate.

We've reached substage seven, the finale.

Substage Seven

All the suffering through the first six stages pales compared to the final stage. Any remaining quality moments are few if at all.

Severest Cognitive Decline

In the seventh stage, daily functions become impossible. Other than an exception here and there, a person cannot recognize anybody. This stage cripples the mind and body and destroys one's ability to talk or communicate.

By this stage, they require 24/7 care and require help with every activity, including going to the bathroom. This stage is why we must prevent this awful disease, for the victim becomes a shell of their former self.

Substage AD Seven Symptoms

- Abnormal reflexes[160]
- Blank facial expressions
- Cannot communicate through words
- Dehydration[161]
- Detached from the surrounding environment
- Groans and moans
- Inability to control bladder

- Inability to control bowel movements
- Infections
- Malnutrition[162]
- Motor skills deteriorate, then disappear
- Pneumonia
- Rigid muscles[163]
- Seizures
- Sleep more
- Unable to breathe
- Unable to sit or hold head up
- Trouble eating or swallowing
- Unable to walk or move (chair or bed bound)
- Weight loss
- people can no longer respond to the surrounding environment[164]

In substage seven, a person requires total care around the clock.

Substage 7 Duration

The duration for the last stage is one to 1.5 to 2.5 years.

Likely Causes of death

There is no substage eight, and substage seven lasts only one to 1.5 years, so this is the final trek of a long and beautiful life.

The causes of death for people carrying Alzheimer's are:

- Dehydration
- Infections
- Malnutrition
- Pneumonia

ALZHEIMER'S STAGES RECAP

We divided Alzheimer's progression into four primary stages, with seven subcategories, which we named stage and substage.

We learned Alzheimer's lingers in the brain for up to twenty years or longer before it manifests, and the first symptoms appear.

In stage one, preclinical Alzheimer's, we learned there are three substages, and the cognitive symptoms are minor but progressing. Because there are no tests, authorities do not consider stage one and its three substages Alzheimer's or dementia.

The first opportunity doctors have with the current system to diagnose Alzheimer's is in stage two and substage four.

The symptoms grow much worse in each stage until they fight the final battle, and the suffering ends.

We learned symptoms present in each stage, and how difficult the disease becomes stages three and four, and impossible during substages five through seven.

Let's review the table below to see how long each stage and substage last.

STAGE	AVERAGE DURATION
1: Preclinical Alzheimer's Substages One	As long as decades
1: Preclinical Alzheimer's Substages Two	Unknown
1: Preclinical Alzheimer's Substages Three	2 to 7 years
2. Early-Stage Alzheimer's Substage Four	2 years
3. Middle-Stage Alzheimer's Substages Five	1.5 years
3. Middle-Stage Alzheimer's Substages Six	2.5 years
4. Late-Stage Alzheimer's Substage Seven	1.5 to 2.5 years

Source: Dementia Care Central[165]

From the time the disease manifests in symptoms, a loved one has five to seventeen years to live once they enter stage two.

They might be a year or two into stage two before being diagnosed, so from that point, the time frame might be shorter.

According to the Mayo Clinic, the average lifespan for somebody with Alzheimer's is between three and 11 years, with some living 20 or more years[166].

Alzheimer's destroys the brain's ability to function, which means the brain, internal organs, and body shut down.

Often, the cause of death will not be Alzheimer's, but something it caused, such as pneumonia, infections, and organ failure.

We hope next year to update this book with breakthroughs in tests, immunizations, and cures. Of the three, testing is likely to be the first breakthrough, but might be two or more years before cleared by the FDA.

Now that we know how typical Alzheimer's progresses, let's see how the atypical or subtypes compare. Keep in mind; the primary differences are in the early stages. In the later stages, the different variants progress similar to typical Alzheimer's.

V. EOAD RELATED RISK FACTORS

This section covers the Alzheimer's-related dementias' risk factors.

As with symptoms and stages, we devote a chapter each to posterior cortical atrophy and LATE, and then a larger chapter covering typical Alzheimer's disease (AD), early-onset Alzheimer's disease (EOAD), and Down syndrome with Alzheimer's disease (DSAD) because they represent three AD manifestation examples and share risk factors.

Chapter 11: EOAD RISK FACTORS

While science does not know the exact cause (s) of Alzheimer's, dozens of studies confirm several Alzheimer's risk factors. Such knowledge points us towards the habits and, sometimes, medicine to avoid or slow Alzheimer's.

While we might discuss overlapping subjects, this short guide's purpose is to provide a simple course on factors within and beyond our control that increases our chances of getting Alzheimer's.

There is another book in the series that focuses on how to prevent or slow Alzheimer's disease. While the books would seem opposites and are, this book is more a prelude to *How to Prevent or Slow Alzheimer's Dementia*. Science might never have figured out steps we can each take to reduce our chances of Alzheimer's, if not for the decades of studies and research that uncovered the risk factors.

While researchers cannot yet find the cause, they have uncovered several risk factors.

There are two risk factors we have no control: Age and genetics (including Down syndrome).

We will examine sixteen total risk factors

1. Age is the obvious risk factor in Alzheimer's dementia.
2. Alcohol Abuse shares similar symptoms and worsens illnesses that elevate one's risk of getting Alzheimer's.
3. Depression is a symptom and a risk factor in Alzheimer's.
4. Diet can protect or destroy our ability to fight diseases such as Alzheimer's as we age.
5. Down Syndrome is a difficult disease that also carries a fifty percent chance of getting Alzheimer's.
6. Genetics blesses and curses us, and one of the cruelest genes point to early-onset Alzheimer's.
7. High Blood Pressure & Hypertension increases one's risk to brain and heart, and Alzheimer's risk.
8. Inactive Minds are a wasteful danger.
9. Low Body Mass does not feed the brain and body and increases one's risk of Alzheimer's.
10. Low Formal Education increases the risk of Alzheimer's unless one educates themselves or otherwise gains an education as an adult.
11. Obesity increases the chances of many devastating diseases, including Alzheimer's.
12. Physical Inactivity, overweight or not, inflates one's chance of heart and brain disease, including Alzheimer's.
13. Prescription Drugs are double-edged swords. While the right medicine can be a lifesaver, the wrong can be

fatal.
14. Sleep Disorders increase the risk of Alzheimer's.
15. Stress boosts the probability of getting Alzheimer's.
16. Tobacco use is a suicidal march, and one of the catastrophic endings is Alzheimer's disease.
17. Type-2 Diabetes is another suicide march toward Alzheimer's.

Age

The older we get, the more at risk we are for Alzheimer's and all adult diseases. Aging itself, however, does not lead to Alzheimer's or memory loss[167].

Since Alzheimer's (not early-onset) strikes those 65 and older, the older one gets, the greater the risk.

A Department of Molecular Neuroscience, Institute of Neurology, University College London concluded: "The greatest risk factor for Alzheimer's disease is advanced age[168]."

None of us can stop the clock, but too many of us complicate the aging process through bad habits.

Everything else we discuss, from factors beyond our control, such as genetics to habits within our control such as diet, affects how we age. Years of neglect, our mind, and bodies carry consequences as we age. Rather than wait until we get older and have problems, we should establish the eating, sleeping, exercising, and positive habits to ward off the preventable dementias and illnesses.

The healthier we eat, the more we exercise, avoid drugs and alcohol, and develop other healthy habits, the less painful and problematic aging must be for each of us. We achieve good health through sacrifice, smart decisions, and work.

In contrast, eating the wrong foods, weak or nonexistent exercise habits, alcohol or drug abuse, and other bad habits catches up with us and makes aging much more complicated than it must be.

For reasons stated, we list age as a related-risk factor for every disease we examine. It is a repetition worth stressing, for even the healthiest and mightiest are mortals.

We'll reiterate the benefits of positive habits and the consequences of bad habits for aging and health.

Alcohol Abuse

When somebody goes to a doctor with Alzheimer's, they will ask if the person drinks alcohol and how much.

Alcohol's relationship to Alzheimer's remains dubious, but alcohol abuse leads to similar cognitive decline symptoms as Alzheimer's. It also can affect blood pressure and diabetes, two known Alzheimer's risk factors.

Alcohol's relationship with tobacco also complicates the effort to determine if alcohol increases one's risk for Alzheimer's.

The Twin Killers

Alcohol and tobacco are the twin killers, for "smokers drink and drinkers smoke[169]."

How many Alcoholics also Smoke Cigarettes?

Between 80 and 95 percent of alcoholics smoke cigarettes, and 70 percent are heavy smokers[170].

Together, alcohol and tobacco synergize, and each inflicts greater harm than they already do by themselves.

There is a chapter on tobacco, but it is important to know the relationship between alcohol and tobacco. Since abusers use alcohol and tobacco, they work together to destroy the mind and body.

How many Americans die each year because of alcohol?

The CDC attributes "88,000 deaths and 2.5 million years of potential life lost[171]," in the United States to alcohol each year.

How many People Worldwide die per year because of Alcohol?

Worldwide, 3.3 million people die from alcohol each year, 5.9 percent of all deaths[172].

Those statistics should provide an incentive not to abuse alcohol. The only smart choices are none and light alcohol consumption. Anything else, including binge drinking, risks major health consequences, including similar symptoms as Alzheimer's.

Science is still unraveling the connection. Researchers work to determine if alcohol abuse causes Alzheimer's.

Does Alcohol Cause Alzheimer's disease?

We know drinking over the limit of one drink per day (females) and two drinks per day (males) increases your odds of getting Alzheimer's and dementia. The more you drink, the higher your risk[173].

According to Alzheimer's Society, drinking over the recommended maximum, even sporadic, "increases a person's risk of developing common types of dementia such as Alzheimer's disease and posterior cortical atrophy [174]."

If you exceed the recommended maximum (one drink for a woman, two for a man) and can't cut back on your own, get help. You're on a self-destructive path you need to get off of as fast as possible for your present and future health.

Prevention Measure # 1

Do not drink alcohol or do not drink over one drink over 24 hours.

If you only drink on the weekend but go over the limit, you put yourself at risk for dementia and many other medical problems.

Some studies suggest one drink for women and two for men is acceptable, some even suggesting health benefits. Other studies label even minimum alcohol consumption unsafe.

All studies confirm any amount over two drinks over any 24 hours is dangerous. Studies also warn binge drinking is almost as dangerous as abusing alcohol every day.

The smart choice: Never drink over one drink over any 24 hours.

The smarter choice: Do not drink alcohol!

Depression

Depression is something everybody suffers to various degrees but, by a 1.7 to 1 ration, women are more likely to suffer the disease[175]. Women's greater prevalence of depression might explain their higher rate of Alzheimer's than men.

The Mayo clinic attributes greater risk of depression to women to what makes them different: Puberty, premenstrual problems, pregnancy, postpartum depression, perimenopause, and menopause, but also point to inequality, working a job and managing the home, sexual and physical abuse[176].

While depression strikes women more often, it does immeasurable damage to both sexes.

Depression is Serious!

Too many suspect depression sufferers exaggerate their symptoms, but others are much worse than suspected. Those with advanced (untreated) depression, suffer more than what most of us experience.

If a loved one becomes depressed, show patience, and do what you can to lift their spirits. If they do not come out of the depression in a reasonable time, or it seems serious, convince them to see a doctor.

Untreated, depression increases our risk of a wide range of serious health issues.

Does Depression cause Alzheimer's?

While researchers debate if depression is the cause or a symptom, they agree it increases one's chances of getting Alzheimer's.

One 28-year study of 10,189 people concluded[177]:

> *Depressive symptoms in the early phase of the study corresponding to midlife, even when chronic/recurring, do not increase the risk for dementia. Along with our analysis of depressive trajectories over 28 years, these results suggest*

that depressive symptoms are a prodromal feature of dementia or that the 2 share common causes. The findings do not support the hypothesis that depressive symptoms increase the risk for dementia.

While the debate continues, there remains no definitive evidence Depression causes Alzheimer's.

A Royal College of Psychiatric study released in the *British Journal of Psychiatry* confirms the results of other studies. Meryl A. Butters, Ph.D., Department of Psychiatry, University of Pittsburg School of Medicine, explained their findings. "Late-life depression," said Butters, "is associated with an increased risk for all-cause dementia, posterior cortical atrophy, and Alzheimer's disease[178]."

Butters calls for: "clinical trials to investigate the effect of late-life depression prevention on risk of dementia, in particular, posterior cortical atrophy and Alzheimer's disease."

Since we know risk factors, it makes sense to study if treating them reduces the risk to Alzheimer's. The government and those with the money should spend the money on the clinical trials Butters and others urge.

Part of Alzheimer's solution might be to treat other diseases such as depression better.

Why is it difficult to distinguish between Alzheimer's & Depression?

In the early and middle stages, Alzheimer's and Depression behavior resemble each other. With no accurate Alzheimer's test, chances of early misdiagnosis remain high.

"Alzheimer's and depression have some similar symptoms," the Mayo Clinic explained. "Proper treatment improves {the} quality of life[179]."

A study supported by the National Institute of Mental Health and the National Institute on Aging confirmed the connection between depression and Alzheimer's and calls for more studies. The researchers explained[180]:

> *The most likely links are the following hypothesized mechanisms: 1) vascular disease; 2) alterations in glucocorticoid steroids and hippocampal atrophy; 3) increased deposition of β-amyloid plaques; 4) inflammatory changes; and 5) deficits of nerve growth factors or neurotrophins.*

Several risk factors, including depression, cause similar brain reactions, symptoms experienced by people carrying Alzheimer's.

Widowed

One late-life form of depression is losing a loved one. Those fortunate enough to find lasting love and both live long lives must face a day when one must live without the other.

Is there anything worse than losing one's soulmate? Of life's many jolts, losing one's life partner is the most difficult for some to overcome, sending them deep into a state of depression, many cannot recover.

When you build your life foundation on a deep partnership with another, losing them is a brutal fate. And, our finite existences means one partner in every meaningful relationship is likely to lose the other at some point.

While many factors are contributing to depression, losing a spouse stands out because often it strikes seniors when they are most vulnerable.

Losing people we love is the worst part of life, and more so for recent widows and widowers.

We need more studies!

Alzheimer's remains mysterious. We don't know if Alzheimer's is Type-3 Diabetes, as some suggest, an outgrowth of Depression, or several important factors.

Scientists from the United States and Europe analyzed several studies on the link between depression and Alzheimer's. "These findings thus underscore the possible relation between the two disorders," they concluded, "and the importance of continued research on the common and disparate factors in the etiology of depression and AD {Alzheimer's disease}[181]."

We reviewed dozens of studies on the link, and everyone emphasized the urgency for new research.

Controlled human studies are also a priority I emphasize throughout our books on Alzheimer's and other dementias.

The human and medical costs of depression and Alzheimer's are too high not to fund the research necessary to cure both. Invest in research now and save money for the government and people over the long run.

We monitor ongoing studies and will update this chapter in our 2020 edition. Please seek treatment for any serious or long term depression.

Prevention Measure #2

Avoid or treat depression. We all get depressed but seek help for severe or prolonged depression.

Living with depression is agony.

Depression also increases our risks for many diseases and links to Alzheimer's and other dementias. We must view severe depression with the same urgency as a broken leg.

Turn to your friends, family, and seek professional help if needed. Like if you had a broken leg, you need help if depression causes you to struggle through each day.

Treat severe depression like the serious medical condition it is. Get help!

In the next section, we examine the diet's relationship to Alzheimer's.

Diet

Nobody likes to discuss our unhealthy diets. We make poor food choices, and we pay the price. If we eat too much, we become congested. If we eat wrong over time, we increase our risk of diseases such as Alzheimer's.

Eating a balanced diet is the best way to remain healthy, but many make horrible food choices. Too much sugar, salt, refined grains, corn syrup. Too little vegetables, fruits, salmon, water,

Whether a meat-eater, vegetarian, or vegan, one can build a tasty, healthy diet. However, too many in each group fail this important task.

We help or hurt ourselves through our food choices. We've already pinpointed diet's importance to the aging process and health.

It's also vital for preventing Alzheimer's. Like the body, if we starve the mind from lack of nutrients, or by poisoning it with the wrong choices, there are consequences, and Alzheimer's and dementia are among the worse.

The Mayo Clinic warns the lack of vegetables and fruit in a diet causes Alzheimer's disease[182].

Processed foods contain dangerous amounts of sweeteners, sodium, preservatives, and harmful chemicals. Food manufacturers remove most of the vitamins, minerals, and nutrients during the processing.

If you eat a poor diet loaded with animal fat and processed foods full of sweeteners and artificial preservatives, you're increasing your chances of Alzheimer's.

Western Diet

Many foods in the Western diet increase Alzheimer's risk. We also know no credible medical researcher ever recommended the Western Diet a medical solution to any symptom or illness.

The Western Diet is a curse that spreads obesity, Type-2 diabetes, hypertension, and other heart and brain illnesses. Eating regular portions would be harmful enough without most of us eating 2-4 times more than our recent ancestors.

Let's review foods you should avoid in the name of longevity.

10 Foods You Should Not Eat or Drink

1. Alcohol (if you drink, do not exceed one drink per day)
2. Diacetyl is a flavoring added to butter, cheese, cookies, candy, crackers, flour, milk, mixes, and microwave popcorn
3. Processed cheese
4. Medication that begins with "anti"
5. Nitrates added to processed and cured meats
6. Processed meats (bacon, deli meat, ham, etc.)
7. Processed foods
8. Smoked meats (including smoked turkey, ham, etc.)
9. White foods (bread, cakes, pasta, rice, etc.)
10. White sugar

As you see, most white foods (other than Cauliflower & white vegetables) are bad for us.

White Poisons

The following are white foods to avoid:
- White flour
- White rice
- White sugar.

The Western diet uses these poisons in abundance in thousands of recipes

Let's review these high-risk foods.

Alcohol

Alcohol might be a risk factor for Alzheimer's disease, but we know heavy drinking worsens the disease. We also know excessive drinking leads or worsens several of the proven risk factors for Alzheimer's: High blood pressure, Type—2 diabetes, and other direct contributors to Alzheimer's. And we know most those who abuse alcohol also are heavy smokers.

Stick to the maximum level (one drink per 24 hours), and you should be okay. If drinking is not important to you, do not drink. Remember, binge drinking (only abusing on weekends or special events) damages our body much like those who abuse alcohol daily.

Diacetyl

Food process companies add Diacetyl as a flavoring to butter, cheese, cookies, candy, crackers, flour, milk, mixes, and popcorn

Medication that begins with "anti"

Avoid the over the counter, and prescribed drugs beginning with "anti" or have "nitrates" in the name.

Nitrates

Manufacturers use nitrates to process and cure meat.

Processed cheese

They process most cheese, and most contain Diacetyl. If you eat cheese, choose aged, non-processed options.

Processed foods

Avoid all processed food. Any healthy diet avoids processed food and focuses on whole food.

Processed meats

Avoid processed meats.

- Bacon
- deli meat
- ham
- other processed meats

Smoked meats

Including smoked turkey, ham, etc.

White foods

Avoid foods using white flour or white sugar:

- bread
- cakes
- pasta
- white rice
- any food made with white flour or white sugar

Instead, eat whole foods that do not require labels. If there is a label with ingredients, there is processing.

White sugar

Do not stock or use white sugar at home. Do not consume sugar-filled drinks and food outside the home.

Prevention Measure 3

Most people control what they eat and drink.

If we eat processed food loaded in sugar and salt, unhealthy habits increase our risk for dementia and several other fatal diseases.

If we eat whole grains, vegetables, wild fish, and a balanced wholefood diet, healthy habits improve our chances for health and prosperity.

We recommend balance and whole foods such as the Mediterranean diet. Whether you are vegan, vegetarian, eat meat, or whatever you call the diet, it boils down to one primary principle.

Eat a balanced wholefood diet!

Down Syndrome

Most of the risk factors outlined in this book are correctable by developing better habits, but not Down syndrome. Genetics only explains five percent of Alzheimer's cases, but those born with Down syndrome are one example.

People with Down syndrome have a third copy of chromosome 21 when two are normal. Research confirms multiple genes in chromosome 21 elevates one's risk for Alzheimer's.

According to the National Down Syndrome Society, people, sixty or older with Down syndrome stand a 50 percent chance of getting Alzheimer's [183].

Those living with Down syndrome carry a thirty percent chance of getting early-onset Alzheimer's[184].

> *Alzheimer's disease affects about 30% of people with Down syndrome in their 50s. By their 60s, this number comes closer to 50%.*

Science has made progress

In the eighties, the life expectancy of those with Down syndrome was under 25 years. Advance three decades and science upped the number beyond sixty[185].

What to do if a loved one has Down syndrome?

See your doctor and follow their advice, or see a new doctor if you do not trust the competency or ethics of the first.

Down Syndrome is not an automatic sentence for Alzheimer's

As the National Down Syndrome Society stresses[186]:

> *While all people with Down syndrome are at risk, many adults with Down syndrome will not manifest the changes of Alzheimer's disease in*

their lifetime. Although risk increases with each decade of life, at no point does it come close to reaching 100%.

We also recommend learning and avoiding the foods and habits that cause Alzheimer's and the dementias and instead eat a whole food diet and practice healthier habits.

Down syndrome is an AD risk factor, no fault of the victims. We hope science soon finds a means to prevent Alzheimer's in 100 percent of people with Down syndrome.

Gender

While scientists have discovered nothing to confirm gender plays a direct role in Alzheimer's development, females make up two-thirds of American Alzheimer's victims[187].

Considering women live longer, we might expect them to suffer a higher rate of disease than men.

Studies suggest; however, women suffer a much higher incidence of Alzheimer's than men, even when accounting for them living longer[188].

Jessica L. Podcasy, MS, and C. Neill Epperson, MD led research on Sex and Gender in Health, University of Pennsylvania Department of Psychiatry explain[189]:

> *Advanced age is the strongest predictor; however, sex and gender differences have been noted in prevalence, clinical manifestation, disease course, and prognosis. Data from the Framingham Study, which enrolled a total of 2611 cognitively intact participants (1550 women and 1061 men) and followed up on many for 20 years, indicated that for a 65-year-old man, remaining lifetime risk of AD was 6.3% (95% confidence interval [CI], 3.9 to 8.7) and remaining lifetime risk of developing any dementing illness was 10.9% (95% CI, 8.0 to 13.8); corresponding risks for a 65-year-old woman were 12% (95% CI, 9.2 to 14.8) and 19% (95% CI, 17.2 to 22.5), almost twice that of men.*

Let's review a study at the University of Luxembourg to see how their results compare.

"Men have a 1 in 11 chance of developing the disease," according to the lead scientist Dr. Enroco Glaab, "but yet for women, the odds are 1 in 6 even when accounting for their longer life span[190]."

The Luxembourg results confirm women are almost twice as likely as men to get Alzheimer's.

From childhood anxiety and depression to childbirth to motherhood, life is never easy for women. But, such unique female hardships do not doom women.

What one eats, how much they exercise, and how one avoids certain things under our control can reduce one's chances.

We need studies comparing healthy women to men who eat unhealthy diets, do not exercise, and are overweight.

My guess is these men with unhealthy habits have a higher chance of Alzheimer's than women who live healthier lifestyles. What we know is women and men can reduce our chances of Alzheimer's by eating healthy, working out, engaging and challenging our minds, and otherwise following scientific advice.

What if Men suffered Alzheimer's the same rates as women?

I am a man, but also a humanist and medical researcher. The men who dominate business and government would devote more money towards Alzheimer's and dementia research if the disease struck middle-aged men instead of older women.

The lengths our leaders go to send young Americans to the other side of the world to launch a war we should not fight should get the politicians thrown out of office. So should their reluctance to invest in legitimate medical research, and their lesser interest in research that benefits women in greater numbers offend humanity.

Sorry for the outburst. Beller Health books are for everybody, no matter one's politics, religion, race, gender, or any other division. The research and books for this book series are apolitical. We follow the research and science and hold no hidden agenda. There is no room for partisanship, bias, or anything else that corrupts research. Our goal is to promote and defend impartial scientific research and to analyze and report the findings.

Can everybody agree our politicians and leaders hold misplaced priorities? When I call them out, it is not a partisan attack, for I could not care less about which party they come. When engaged in this book, my colleagues and I place victims, cures, knowledge, symptoms, risks over political party or group identification.

Here, as a male medical researcher, it is clear women do not always receive equal medical attention as men, and the gap grows more pronounced with minority females.

My colleagues and I call for greater funding into Alzheimer's research, and specific studies to identify why women are twice as likely to carry Alzheimer's as men.

Does genetics explain the greater Alzheimer's prevalence in women?

Genetics might play a role, but environmental factors such as women's products uncommon for men also might explain the disparity. It is inconclusive.

Genetics

Genetics causes less than five percent of Alzheimer's cases. [191] Science has found several genes that increase the odds but do not guarantee one gets Alzheimer's. If a parent or sibling has the disease, it increases one's chances of Alzheimer's.

Dozens of large studies over 30 years reviewed[192]:

> To date, more than 20 non-APOE-related loci exhibit {a} nominally significant association with disease risk in systematic meta-analyses of the available AD genetic literature7. These findings implicate many of the potential culprits that have long been believed to be involved in the development of neurodegeneration and dementia (such as APP metabolism, Ab degradation and clearance, signal transduction, tau dysfunction, protein trafficking, cholinergic deficits, cholesterol metabolism and the homeostasis of heavy metals).

Genetic Relation to Early-onset Alzheimer's

Genetics plays a large role in early-onset, which accounts for less than ten percent of Alzheimer's.

How many Americans have early-onset Alzheimer's?

Of the 5.5 million Americans with Alzheimer's, over 200,000 have early-onset[193].

How do parents weigh into the equation?

"A child whose biological mother or father carries a genetic mutation for early-onset FAD has a 50/50 chance of inheriting that mutation," reported the National Institute on Aging. "If the mutation is inherited, the child has a very strong probability of developing early-onset FAD[194]."

Each parent or sibling with Alzheimer's increases your chances of getting the disease.

However, Alzheimer's threatens all humans, and we all have the same prevention plan. What we control is establishing good habits and reducing our bad habits that increase our chances of getting Alzheimer's.

The next step

The next step is to find a means to stop the risk genes in their tracks. A study released in *Nature Medicine* is one of the more promising because it used human genes, instead of testing on lab rats.

The Gladstone Institutes study lead author Yadong Huang explained the importance. "Drug development for Alzheimer's disease has been largely a disappointment over the past ten years," said Huang. "Many drugs work beautifully in a mouse model, but so far they've all failed in clinical trials. One concern within the field has been how poorly these mouse models mimic human disease[195]."

While animal testing has helped advance medicine, what works on rats might not work on humans. The Gladstone Institutes scientists in the *Nature Medicine* study discovered how apoE4 increases the risk of Alzheimer's. More importantly, the scientists devised a way to convert it into a "harmless apoE3-like version[196]."

While scientists must conduct more studies before we see any such treatment available to the public, such breakthroughs might one day provide a godsend for those who carry the risk genes.

High Blood Pressure And Hypertension

For most people, bad habits lead to high blood pressure and hypertension, raising the risk of heart disease and Alzheimer's. Not to shame anybody, but we humans accumulate bad habits, which have consequences, and one is high blood pressure.

We examine how high blood pressure increases Alzheimer's risks.

How does high blood pressure increase Alzheimer's risks?

Studies suggest high blood pressure inhibits the protein ACE, which breaks down the harmful amyloid protein associated with Alzheimer's.

American Academy of Neurology Study

A study published in the *American Academy of Neurology* followed 1,288 people, 65 percent women, and found Alzheimer's "pathology showed an association of a higher mean SBP with a higher number of tangles[197]."

Funded by the National Institutes of Health, study author Zoe Arvanitakis, MD, MS, of the Rush Alzheimer's Disease Center at Rush University Medical Center in Chicago said reported high systolic blood pressure increases the risk of brain lesions by 46 percent or more.

"When looking for signs of Alzheimer's disease in the brain at autopsy," Arvanitakis said, "researchers found a link between higher average late-life systolic blood pressure across the years before death and a higher number of tangles[198]."

How is blood pressure measured?

We gauge blood pressure by measuring two pressures, systolic (top number) and diastolic (bottom number).

Systolic Pressure

Systolic pressure measures artery and blood vessels pressure per heartbeat.

Diastolic Pressure

Diastolic pressure measures the pressure between heartbeats.

What is normal blood pressure, high blood pressure, and hypertension?

New Blood Pressure Reading Measurements

The American Heart Association established new guidelines for blood pressure readings. Let's review the chart of their updated recommendations:

BP Category	Systolic BP		Diastolic BP
Normal	<120 mmHg	and	<80 mmHg
Elevated	120-129 mmHg	and	<80 mmHg
Hypertension: stage 1	130-139 mmHg	or	80-89 mmHg
Hypertension: stage 2	≥140 mmHg	or	≥90 mmHg
Hypertensive emergency	>180 mmHg	and/or + target organ damage	>120 mmHg

Source: American College of Cardiology/American Heart Association Task Force on Clinical Practice Guidelines[199].

The new guidelines lower the maximum normal, elevated,

and hypertension blood pressure levels.

High Blood Pressure

How many people have high blood pressure?

United States

In another indictment of the modern Western diet and lifestyle, the American Heart Association claims 103 million, almost half of American adults, have high blood pressure or hypertension.

According to Dr. Paul Muntner, co-chair of the American Heart Association report, the updated numbers are but the start of bad news. "With the aging of the population and increased life expectancy," said Muntner, "the prevalence of high blood pressure is expected to continue to increase[200]."

Worldwide

World Health Organization reports high blood pressure causes 7.5 million deaths, 12.8 percent of annual fatalities, and that one billion people live with untreated hypertension[201].

The silent killer

High blood pressure is known as the silent killer because, much like Alzheimer's, it shows no outward symptoms in the earlier stages.

What causes high blood pressure?

Age

Despite our protests, the older we reach, the greater our risks to high blood pressure, heart disease, and Alzheimer's.

Alcohol abuse

If we drink over one drink per 24 hour period, we risk serious consequences, and high blood pressure is one.

Excess salt (sodium)

Most fast and restaurant food has too much salt, as does

canned foods. Despite food already too salted, the first thing the average person does when the food arrives is dash or shovel more salt.

Overloading sodium is a deadly habit.

Family history

A family history of blood pressure increases our risks. Genetics might play a role in rare cases, but bad habits cause high blood pressure and pass along within families.

Illegal drugs

Many illegal drugs cause significant health risks. Different drugs attack specific areas of the body and mind. One side effect of certain illegal drug use is high blood pressure.

Other medical conditions

Diabetes, kidney disease, and sleep apnea elevate blood pressure.

Overweight or obesity

Being overweight leads to diabetes and high blood pressure.

Physical inactivity

Related to being overweight is physical inactivity.

Prescribed Medication

I want to be the first to salute modern medicine for the many breakthroughs that extend and improve our lives, but—because of an inadequate health care system—the average doctor writes prescriptions faster than the best illegal drug dealer can unload their product.

Some medication is a godsend, while the other is a demon-send, for the side effects too often offset any potential benefit.

Race

African Americans are much more likely to get high blood pressure than the rest of the population.

Stress

Continuous or critical stress can lead to anxiety and high blood pressure. While minimizing and controlling stress is easier said than done, it might save our lives.

Tobacco

Of the million reasons to avoid tobacco, it increases the risk of high blood pressure.

Too little potassium

Related to high levels of salt (sodium), the Western Diet has too little potassium. Avoiding or combatting high blood pressure require we consume more potassium in our foods than sodium. Instead, most American foods are high in sodium and low in potassium.

Prevention Measure 3

To avoid strokes, vascular disease, and dementia, one must control their blood pressure.

If you have or want to avoid high blood pressure, please include the following eight recommendations:

1. Improve your diet by eating more fruit, vegetables, and whole grains[202].
2. Exercise. Run, walk, swim, hike, whatever you will do several times per week.
3. If you use any tobacco product, stop!
4. Minimize stress. We all experience stress, but we control how we respond.
5. If you are overweight, combine a diet and exercise plan that will help reduce it to an acceptable level.
6. Try to build a three to one ratio of potassium to sodium in your diet.
7. If you drink alcohol, limit it to one drink per 24 hours.
8. If you use illegal drugs, stop.

Inactive Mind

As dangerous as a dormant body is an inactive mind.

Our ancestors traveled by foot and did everything by hand, so they received continuous physical exercise. If they hoped for longevity, their minds focused on finding food and shelter and avoiding hostile animals and humans. Survivors among our ancestors did so because they developed and practiced the physical and mental habits to survive.

Modern humans spend too much time sitting at work, then on the sofa watching television in the evening. The combination of inactivity and poor diets do not provide the brain stimuli needed for growth. Unhealthy diets starve the brain of important nutrients, while not exercising our brian allows it to weaken like any neglected muscle.

Half of Americans have high blood pressure and are overweight, a combination lowering the human physical and cognitive potential. We know how to eat healthier, engage in brain stimuli, and develop our bodies in ways our ancestors could not have fathomed.

Yet half of Americans, and a similar number of global citizens, scoff at the information and tools and instead pursue a life of indulgence, recklessness, and unnecessary danger. We are stubborn!

How is Brain Exercise related to Alzheimer's?

A study released in the *American Academy of Neurology* concluded[203]:

> *How often older people read a newspaper, play chess, or engage in other mentally stimulating activities is related to {the} risk of developing Alzheimer's disease, according to a new study. The study found a cognitively active person in old age was 2.6 times less likely to develop dementia and Alzheimer's disease than a*

cognitively inactive person in old age. This association remained after controlling for past cognitive activity, lifetime socioeconomic status, and current social and physical activity.

A study in the Journal of the American Medical Association analyzed 801 older priests, brothers, and nuns. Robert S. Wilson, Ph.D., and the team found: "frequent participation in cognitively stimulating activities is associated with reduced risk of AD[204]."

Prevention Measure 4

Exercise your brain! Free, challenge, engage, and stimulate your mind! As the *Swiss Medical Weekly* says of cognitive activity, "Use it or lose it[205]."

Among the recommended cognitive activity:

- Keep learning. Learn a new language. Study history. The important thing is to keep learning, which expands the mind
- Play games, thinking games like chess
- Read books
- Write a diary
- Write letters
- Read a credible daily newspaper (or ten or twenty online)
- Attend a social function
- Call (or better visit) family and friends

Challenging the mind is rewarding and fun. History, art, science, nature, and several avenues provide fabulous brain exercise. Pursue things that inspire, move, challenge, and feeds your passion and mind.

Low Formal Education

The lower the level of formal education, the higher one's Alzheimer's risk.

I do not believe formal education is necessary, but education is the key.

Three of the great American presidents were self-taught men. Those three men—Abe Lincoln, Harry Truman, and Dwight Eisenhower—are three of our most revered presidents.

The one thing the three had in common is they read and worked harder to learn than their counterparts who received formal education.

My point is one can always read. If you cannot read, turn to somebody who will teach you and spend the rest of your life reading.

The University of Southern California, Department of Psychology Research

A University of Southern California team analyzed 88 studies and 71 articles to determine if lower education levels increased risks of Alzheimer's. "Lower education was associated with a greater risk for dementia in many but not all studies," reported Margaret Gatz, Ph.D. "Of the 13 studies that analyzed the relationship between low education and risk for AD, seven studies reported significant effects such that lower education was associated with an increased risk for AD."

Study Released in the American Journal of Epidemiology

A study released in the *American Journal of Epidemiology* found a lower a woman's educational level, the higher their risks of Alzheimer's[206].

Study Published in the Medical Journal for the American Academy of Neurology

A study from Finland published in the American Academy of Neurology followed almost 1,400 people for 21 years. They found[207]:

> *People who don't finish high school are at a higher risk of developing dementia and Alzheimer's disease compared to people with more education, regardless of lifestyle choices and characteristics such as income, occupation, physical activity, and smoking,*

University of Cambridge Study

A team of researchers from the UK and Finland examined the brains of 872 who took part in three large aging studies, so their past was well-documented.

"Over the past decade, studies on dementia have consistently showed that the more time you spend in education, the lower your risk of dementia," said co-author Dr. Hannah Keage of the University of Cambridge. "For each additional year of education, there is an 11% decrease in risk of developing dementia."

There appears to be a link to educational level and Alzheimer's, but again I caution not to paint with too broad of a brush. Those with lower education levels also make less money, receive inferior health care, live in homes and neighborhoods that pose greater health risks, and face a different norm than do the middle or upper classes.

I believe education matters, whether it be formal. If a person reads, writes, thinks, engages their mind, avoids trouble, minimizes stress, enjoys life, knows history, embraces science, and practices the Golden Rule, they will overcome their lack of formal education.

Prevention Measure 4

Reversing the risk is not a matter of hanging a fancy diploma on the wall, but about challenging and exercising your mind, the same thing we recommended for the inactive mind risk.

Although enrolling at a community college (or four-year school) is a great option, learning is the key.

This world is a great adventure. Study the stars. Learn a new skill. Study the world around you. Keep a journal. Play chess. Read books. Write poetry. Develop art. Learn! Learn! Learn! Every single day of your life!

Obesity

Like the rest of the book, his section is not about shame. By the time we reach forty, most of us are battling body fat and more so with the past couple generations where the average person has eaten more and exercised less.

Type-2 Diabetes is a serious disease that leads to a variety of other, even worse, diseases. Here's the difference between Type-2 Diabetes and the average killer disease; Type-2 Diabetes results from almost 100 percent eating too large of helpings of the wrong food, and engaging in too little physical exercise.

Also related to diet and exercise is obesity, which leads to Type-2 Diabetes, which causes strokes, which leads to Alzheimer's disease[208].

Obesity is the front and center of contemporary health issues. If you want to avoid Alzheimer's and other severe illnesses, it's vital to control your weight.

Study Published in the United States Library of Medicine National Institutes of Health

A group of scientists reviewed longitudinal epidemiological studies to determine obesity and diabetes' risk factors for Alzheimer's. They concluded: "Obesity and diabetes significantly and independently increase risk for AD[209]."

A Second Study Published in the United States Library of Medicine National Institute of Health

The study followed 10,276 women and men for almost ten years to determine the relationship between obesity and Alzheimer's. They concluded: "Obesity in middle age increases the risk of future dementia independently of comorbid conditions[210]."

A Third Study Published in the Journal of the American Medical Association

The Cardiovascular Risk Factors, Aging, and Dementia Study analyzed studies from 1972 to 1987, then recruited 1,449 people for an average 21-year follow-up examination. They concluded: "Obesity at midlife is associated with an increased risk of dementia and AD later in life[211]."

The evidence appears clear that obesity increases the risks of Alzheimer's (and several other diseases). If you or loved ones are overweight, please take steps to reduce your weight within the excepted weight range for your height and gender.

Weight is something ninety-plus percent of us can defeat with a solid plan and will power. It will not be easy but will be one of your greatest personal accomplishments, and among your proudest.

Physical Inactivity

Related to obesity is physical inactivity. The average American (human) consumes too much food, and the only way to balance the extra calories is to remain active.

The modern world offers an abundance of food for anybody who can afford, and a variety of movies, television series, social media options, and other gadgets that park one in a seat for hours.

If we follow every fad, we all end up with a weight problem, which leads to Type-2 diabetes, which increases the risks for cancer, heart attacks, strokes, Alzheimer's, and other dementias.

Study Released in the Journal of the American Medical Association

A New York study followed 1,880 people without dementia over 15 years. "In this study," said Nikolaos Scarmeas, MD, "both higher Mediterranean-type diet adherence and higher physical activity were independently associated with reduced risk for AD[212]."

Systematic Review of Several Studies

This systematic review found physical inactivity increased cognitive decline risk in 20 of 24 longitudinal studies[213].

A Second Systematic Review of Several Studies

These scientists and researchers analyzed dozens of studies. They concluded[214]:

> The majority of longitudinal epidemiological studies have clearly shown associations between physical activities and the risk of cognitive decline in a dose-response manner suggesting

that physical activities may delay the onset of AD as well as the risk of cognitive decline and mortality.

Our bodies break down when we do not engage ourselves in continuous physical activity. Not getting enough exercise is as bad for our minds as our bodies.

Prevention Measure 5

Walk. Swim. Run. Hike. These and other physical activities strengthen your body and mind and reduce your chances of Alzheimer's.

Also, lift light weights or perform resistance exercises three days per week.

If you enjoy life, take steps to enhance health and longevity. Be active!

Prescription Drugs

According to Science Daily, "Multiple drug classes commonly prescribed for common medical conditions are capable of influencing the onset and progression of Alzheimer's disease[215]."

A Harvard study warns that benzodiazepines increase the risk of Alzheimer's and poses the greatest risk to older people[216].

We require more tests on the long-range effects of benzodiazepines and other prescription drugs. While we might know the short-term effects of some of these drugs, they conduct too few studies to determine their long-term consequences.

Harvard Medical School reviewed two studies[217]:

> *In two separate large population studies, both benzodiazepines (a category that includes medications for anxiety and sleeping pills) and anticholinergics (a group that encompasses medications for allergies and colds, depression, high blood pressure, and incontinence) were associated with an increased risk of dementia in people who used them for longer than a few months. In both cases, the effect increased with the dose of the drug and the duration of use.*

These drugs are dangerous and in many prescription and over-the-counter drugs. There have not been enough long-term studies for thousands of other drugs to know if they increase Alzheimer's risks (or other serious health risks).

A Review Published in the British Medical Journal

This review focused on 300,000 seniors, their medical use, and the risks of Alzheimer's and other dementias. They found those who took medication containing anticholinergic increased their risk of Alzheimer's and other dementias by a minimum of 11 percent. The number rose to 30 percent for those who consumed the most anticholinergic[218].

Worst Pills

Worst Pills, Best Pills lists 136 drugs that cause cognitive impairment, including drug-induced dementia. Their list includes most of the drugs linked to a greater risk of Alzheimer's, including anticholinergic, benzodiazepines, eszopiclone, opiates, zolpidem (AMBIEN), zaleplon, sedatives, tricyclic antidepressants[219].

If your doctor prescribes any medication, check to see if the drugs contain any of the above. Make certain your doctor knows of the higher risks of Alzheimer's and other dementias and ask if taking the medication is worth the risk.

Also, watch out for any of these ingredients in over-the-counter drugs. Better yet, try to avoid most over-the-counter drugs. Most get credit for illnesses that go away on their own and have dozens of side effects worse than the modest symptoms they claim to cure.

A Broken System

The problem with the average drug dealer, legal or illegal, is they place profit over their fellow human being's welfare.

Big Pharmaceutical

Pharmaceutical is in business (like those in other industries) to make a profit. Anybody who works for a corporation knows corporate (and board members) profits are the priority. For this discussion, the statement is a fact and does not weigh in on the ethics. My point is they are there to profit, not for the public good.

Insurance Companies

Most people have sorry insurance. The average Americans choose from "insurance" options resembling fool's gold. Expensive premiums, high deductibles, and low coverage are bankrupting American families and a drag on the national and global economy.

The Affordable Care Act

A half-baked plan intended to evolve into real insurance, the Affordable Care Act has stagnated in Congress and remains nothing more than catastrophic coverage forced on those who cannot afford it, and does little to help them with health care.

Congress

The political parties must advance the coverage into real insurance like Congress did Social Security.

Democrats must admit the Affordable Care Act does not provide Americans legitimate and affordable insurance, and Republicans need to help improve the Affordable Care Act or offer an alternative proposal (something they did not do in all this time they complained and sabotaged the Affordable Care Act). Everybody in Congress should be ashamed of forcing poor people to buy catastrophic insurance dressed up as medical coverage. The poor cannot afford $10,000 deductibles before any coverage kicks in!

I call on Congress and politicians around the world to take Alzheimer's, dementia, and people's health care serious. Stop playing political soccer and using people's health as your ball.

Lower the costs and improve the coverage for all people!

Doctors

General practitioners today fight to remain in business like everybody else and sorry insurance policies has turned the typical doctor visit into:

- Fill out a lot of paperwork you have already filled out (in the digital age!)
- Camp in the waiting room for up to an hour or more
- A nurse takes you to a room and perhaps takes your blood pressure and asks you a few questions like what are your symptoms
- Wait in the room for another fifteen minutes or longer before the doctor arrives
- The doctor spends five minutes with you and writes one or more prescriptions

Doctors write too many prescriptions, and Americans consume too many legal and illegal drugs. If required, medications work right and do not cause a reaction worse than what they are curing, and we endorse such prescriptions 100 percent.

But, the herd them in and out medical system in the United States and most the world does not allow doctors to get to know their patients, learn their full symptoms, or to counsel them on safer, natural options that work as well or better than some of these drugs.

To herd them through like sorry health insurance demands,

and to prevent getting sued, doctors write prescriptions only five minutes after seeing a patient. The continuous prescriptions allow doctors to claim they treated symptoms, and moves you along to the pharmacy to fill your prescriptions, as the pharmaceutical companies demand.

The doctor, Big Pharmaceutical, and insurance companies get paid, while the patient too often gets the shaft.

If doctors are okay with getting paid and looking the other way, continue as usual. If you want more than our medical system offers, speak out!

Prevention Measure 6

Do yourself a favor and avoid or minimize prescription drugs. But how?

What is a person to do?

Be proactive. Eat right, exercise, avoid stress, and do what we must to achieve ultimate health.

Whether you are one of the fortunate with quality medical insurance and care or one of the many with bad or no coverage, our best option is to feed and exercise our bodies and minds like we deserve. Otherwise, we are cheating ourselves.

If you are sick, listen to your doctor, but ask about a prescription's side effect or if there is a natural alternative treatment that would work as well or better. If you take medication, do not take more than the prescription dictates. Remember, avoiding long term use of any medication is best, so try to take natural steps to get off the medication as soon as possible.

Closing Note

Do not stop taking any medication you are already taking without consulting your doctor. If you have a problem requiring medication and your doctor prescribes it, take as directed.

Minimize it!

Sleep Disorder

We need our sleep, so our body and mind can cleanse and reboot for the next grueling 16 or 17 hours. Humans require 7-8 hours of sleep, and as much deep-sleep as possible.

Many things keep us up at night. Stress. Depression. Guilty conscience. Fears. Jealousies. Spite. We eat the wrong foods, too close to bedtime. Allergies and dozens of other diseases keep us awake when we should be sleeping.

Even if nothing is wrong with us, there are trains, automobiles, airplanes, neighbors, and other modern noises that deprive us of valuable sleep. Our challenge is to overcome the noise pollution and get sleep.

Dr. Ronald Petersen, Alzheimer's Disease Research Center, Mayo Clinic, Rochester, Minnesota, investigated sleep apnea's link to Alzheimer's.

"Not only could long-term sleep deprivation raise your risk for dementia {Alzheimer's}," said Dr. Peterson, "research has shown that, over time, people who don't sleep enough also may be at an increased risk for other health problems, including high blood pressure, heart disease, and diabetes[220]."

Note that high blood pressure, heart disease, and diabetes also increase the risks of Alzheimer's.

Tests suggest sleep apnea increases the risk of Alzheimer's by developing a higher level of beta-amyloid protein than those who sleep well.

Let's review if sleep apnea increases the risk of Alzheimer's.

New York University School of Medicine

A New York University School of Medicine study found that 30 to 80 percent of seniors experience sleep apnea. "Those with sleep apnea accumulated amyloid plaque," explained study spokesperson Dr. Ricardo Osorio, "which could trigger

Alzheimer's in the future[221]."

A Review in Science Direct

A *Science Direct* study probed dozens of studies and concluded: "Clinical studies suggest an increased incidence of Alzheimer's disease in sleep apnea patients[222]."

University of California Study

Another University of California study released in the *Journal of the American Medical Association* focused on older women in their eighties. The study concluded those suffering sleep apneas were twice as likely to develop Alzheimer's or another dementia in the next five years as those who slept uninhibited[223].

The studies are consistent that sleep apnea causes cognitive impairment and increases the chance of Alzheimer's and the dementias.

Prevention Measure 7

Too many people consider sleep optional. Others suffer medical issues that inhibit sleep. Both increases risk for dozens of fatal disorders, including Alzheimer's and several dementias.

We recommend you get one of the watch-like devices and monitor your sleep to measure your total sleep and deep sleep. A person requires seven to eight hours of sleep per night, and as much deep sleep as possible.

If you are not getting enough sleep, you might feel sleepy during the day. Trouble remaining awake during the day is a warning sign, so take it seriously.

A few pointers.

- Establish firm times to go to bed and get up.
- Avoid alcohol
- Do not eat spicy foods.
- Avoid any habits, foods, or activities that keep you up at night.
- Use white noise to minimize noise pollution
- Meditate

You must sleep without sleeping pills, which cause too many side effects. Try the listed recommendations and otherwise search for natural means to enhance your sleep.

Get seven to eight hours sleep; no more, no less.

Stress

Follow Bobby McFerrin's advice: Don't worry, be happy[224]. Stress kills humans and raises your risks to Alzheimer's[225].

Unmanaged stress causes anxiety, attacking your insides for months, years, or even decades. Stress and anxiety cause a high rate of Beta-amyloid plaque.

Why is Beta-amyloid a problem?

Beta-amyloid

Let's turn to Director Christopher Rowe of the nuclear medicine department and Center for PET at Austin Hospital in Melbourne, Victoria, Australia. The Australian team studied Beta-amyloid.

"Beta-amyloid is associated with brain dysfunction - even in apparently normal elderly individuals," said Rowe, "providing further evidence it is likely related to the fundamental cause of Alzheimer's disease[226]."

How do Studies Connect Stress to Alzheimer's?

Let's review a few studies and reviews to determine stress's relationship to Alzheimer's.

Wisconsin School of Medicine Review

One of the interesting presentations at the *Alzheimer's Association International Conference* in London was a Wisconsin School of Medicine test measuring stress's relationship to Alzheimer's. The researchers studied 1,320 people[227]:

> *Every stressful event was equal to 1.5 years of brain aging across all participants, except for African-Americans, where every stressful event was equal to 4 years of brain aging.*

That is horrible news for everybody, and numbers African-Americans should pay particular attention. When people say stress is a killer, they are not joking. We plan a book on the added stress factor for African-Americans, Native-Americans (ones here when the Europeans arrived), other minorities, and poor of every type, including European descendants. Most Americans stress, but those at the bottom must carry an even greater load.

The University of Wisconsin study: "concluded that the participants from the most disadvantaged areas performed worse in every aspect of cognitive testing and had higher levels of biomarkers for Alzheimer's."

Those climbing from the bottom face many stressful obstacles, causing constant and severe stress. All classes of modern humans stress, the consequences often are fatal, so we must learn to reduce stress, avoid it when possible, and otherwise minimize.

Let's turn to some other studies and reviews to determine how stress increases the risks of Alzheimer's.

Review Published in Current Opinion in Psychiatry

The lead author, Dr. Linda Mah, Department of Psychiatry, University of Toronto, and team reviewed several large studies.

"Pathological anxiety and chronic stress are associated with structural degeneration and impaired functioning of the hippocampus and the prefrontal cortex," said Dr. Mah, "which may account for the increased risk of developing neuropsychiatric disorders, including depression and dementia {Alzheimer's}[228]."

Chronic stress is dangerous but leads to a greater threat, anxiety. In the classroom, workplace, traffic, lines at stores, and in the comfort of one's home, minimizing stress should be a top priority. We can blow our top dozens of times per day in the modern rat race.

Don't do it!

Moody, Jealous, Worrisome Women have Higher Alzheimer's Risk

A study published in the American Academy of Neurology followed 800 women for 38 years to determine if stress increased their risk of Alzheimer's. Lead author Lena Johansson, Ph.D., at the University of Gothenburg, spoke for the group of researchers.

"Women who are anxious, jealous, or moody and distressed in middle age," Johansson said, "may be at a higher risk of developing Alzheimer's disease later in life[229]."

Although the study only tested women, other studies suggest men also carry a higher risk of Alzheimer's if they worry too much, are moody, or always jealous about something or someone.

Men and women must reduce the stress in our lives and lessen our risks to Alzheimer's, other dementias, and fatal health issues.

Prevention Measure 8

How important is managing stress?
Let's turn to Harvard Medical School.

Harvard Medical School

"Stress management may reduce health problems linked to stress, which include cognitive problems and a higher risk for Alzheimer's disease and dementia[230]."

Managing stress might save your life and help you avoid dementia. A few recommendations:

- Meditation
- Exercise each day
- Eat a balanced wholefood diet
- Avoid people and activities that cause your stress

Take these and other natural steps to reduce your stress, improve your health, and increase your longevity.

Tobacco

Tobacco has killed more humans than all wars combined. For the killer weed, politicians and business people have always placed profit above public safety.

Using tobacco increases your risk of almost every disease on the planet, including Alzheimer's disease. Both smoking and secondhand smoke cause Alzheimer's[231].

Tobacco is a senseless habit that has killed more people than all wars combined.

"The chief preventable cause of death worldwide," says the World Alzheimer's Report[232].

> The annual global deaths due to tobacco are still expected to increase from the current six million, to eight million people by 2030. Cigarette smoking is causally related to a wide range of diseases 42 including many forms of cancer, cardiovascular disease and diabetes as well as increased risk of dyslipidaemia. The most prevalent dementia subtypes, vascular dementia (VaD) and Alzheimer's disease (AD), have been linked to underlying vascular mechanisms and neurovascular events.

Tobacco addiction makes a person crave and feel they cannot live without an immediate fix, but it destroys the body and mind.

Secondhand smoke also increases your risk for many diseases, so do not allow others to smoke in your presence, or in any establishment you live, work, or frequent.

How does Tobacco Increase Alzheimer's Risk?

Let's begin with a Columbia University study.

Columbia University Study Published in the US National Library of Medicine National Institutes of Health

A Columbia University study followed 1,138 dementia-free people in their seventies to determine if smoking tobacco elevates risks of Alzheimer's.

The researchers analyzed data from a northern Manhattan longitudinal study and found smoking and diabetes were the highest risk factors for Alzheimer's. They concluded: "Our results are consistent with the observation that smoking increases the risk of AD {Alzheimer's}[233]."

A University of San Francisco Review Published in the US National Library of Medicine National Institutes of Health

The University of San Francisco researchers reviewed several published studies on tobacco and nicotine. They compared smokers to nonsmokers[234].

> The literature indicates that former/active smoking is related to a significantly increased risk for AD. Cigarette smoke/smoking is associated with AD neuropathology in preclinical models and humans. Smoking-related cerebral oxidative stress is a potential mechanism promoting AD pathophysiology and increased risk for AD.

The Observational University of California Study Published on Pub Med

A University of California observational studies found smokers carry a 79 percent greater risk of Alzheimer's than do nonsmokers[235].

World Health Organization

The World Health Organization claims smoking increases

one's chance of Alzheimer's by 45 percent[236].

Every credible organization I know lists tobacco as a risk for Alzheimer's and Posterior cortical atrophy. Nature and man have never built another killer like tobacco, as it kills millions each year, and leaves millions of others with one dementia, cancer, or some other devastating disease.

If you smoke, the best thing you can do for yourself and those around you is to quit. Among other health benefits, it will reduce your risk of Alzheimer's.

Prevention Measure 9

Do not smoke!

If you already smoke, quit! If you do not smoke, never start!

Do not use any tobacco products. No vaping. No cigarettes. No chewing tobacco. No snuff. No tobacco in any recreational form!

Type-2 Diabetes

According to the American Diabetes Association, 9.4 percent of Americans, over 30 million in total, have diabetes[237].

Let's review the global population.

The World Health Organization (WHO) reports that over 422 million people have Type-2 diabetes worldwide[238]. WHO lists Type-2 diabetes as the seventh leading cause of death worldwide, two behind Alzheimer's disease at number five[239].

Worldwide, a minimum of 371 million people has Type-2 diabetes.

Type-2 Diabetes is 100 percent Avoidable!

Type-2 diabetes is 100 percent avoidable, and fixable through diet, exercise, and weight management.

Before high blood sugar elevates enough to Type-2 Diabetes levels, there is a period called Hyperglycemia/high blood sugar/prediabetes.

Before we dive into Type-2 Diabetes, let's determine if prediabetes increases the risk of Alzheimer's.

High Blood Sugar/Hyperglycemia/Prediabetes

Hyperglycemia, meaning high blood sugar, but not high enough to rank as diabetes. For this discussion, we refer to it as prediabetes.

Several studies link high blood sugar levels and higher Alzheimer's risks, speeding and worsening the disease.

Let's begin with a German study that changed the way we view blood sugar and how the brain processes it.

Director of the drug discovery division at the German Center for Diabetes Research (DZD), Matthias Tschöp reported their findings[240]:

Our results showed for the first time that essential metabolic and behavioral processes are not regulated via neuronal cells alone and that other cell types in the brain, such as astrocytes, play a crucial role. This represents a paradigm shift and could help explain why it has been so difficult to find sufficiently efficient and save medicines for diabetes and obesity until now.

While other studies had discovered a link between high blood pressure and Alzheimer's, the German study might explain why. We now know much more is going on inside the brain than we thought when processing sugar.

Type-2 Diabetes

If prediabetes elevates the risks of Alzheimer's, Type-2 Diabetes is a bigger culprit. Type-2 diabetes, obesity, high blood pressure each to varying degrees the product of poor diets, and inadequate exercise.

An obese person has a higher risk of developing Type-2 diabetes and hypertension. The three diseases attack cells and damage the brain, heart, and blood flow.

Obesity, high blood pressure, and Type-2 diabetes is the perfect cocktail for strokes, heart disease, and the dementias, including Alzheimer's.

Studies confirming Type-2 Diabetes link to Alzheimer's

Scientists at the University of Cambridge teamed up with colleagues in Taiwan and Japan to follow 67,731 participants to study the connection. "Diabetes is associated with an increased risk of dementia[241]," reported Stephen Kritchevsky, Ph.D.

Early diagnosis and the correct medication can offset the risk. "The risk effect becomes weaker," said Kritchevsky said, "provided that participants take sulfonylureas or metformin rather than thiazolidinedione for a longer period."

Researchers in another longitudinal cohort study followed

824 older priests, brothers, and nuns in annual examinations over nine years. They concluded diabetes mellitus raised Alzheimer's risks and caused cognitive function decline in older persons[242]:

> *Diabetes mellitus was present in 127 (15.4%) of the participants. During a mean of 5.5 years of observation, 151 persons developed AD. In a proportional hazards model adjusted for age, sex, and educational level, those with diabetes mellitus had a 65% increase in the risk of developing AD compared with those without diabetes mellitus (hazard ratio, 1.65; 95% confidence interval, 1.10-2.47). In random effects models, diabetes mellitus was associated with lower levels of global cognition, episodic memory, semantic memory, working memory, and visuospatial ability at baseline. Diabetes mellitus was associated with a 44% greater rate of decline in perceptual speed (P = .02), but not in other cognitive systems.*

Most research confirms Type-2 diabetes increases risks to Alzheimer's by 50 to 65 percent.

How about when Diabetes Patients also experience Depression?

A University of Washington School of Medicine study focused on 19,239 diabetes patients to determine if diabetes and depression carried extra Alzheimer's risks. Wayne Katon, MD, Professor and Vice-Chair, Department of Psychiatry & Behavioral Sciences, reported their findings.

"Depression in patients with diabetes," said Katon, "with a substantively increased risk for development of dementia compared to those with diabetes alone[243]."

Depression compounds other diseases, including diabetes, hypertension, obesity, intensifying Alzheimer's risk factors for each.

Prevention Measure 10

Through bad habits, we cause most type-2 diabetes. Our recommendations to avoid type-2 diabetes:

- A balanced wholefood diet
- Daily exercise
- Avoid sitting for longer than 25 minutes
- Do not drink alcohol

VI. BONUS SECTION

Whether diagnosed with dementia or preparing for a rainy day, there are basics everybody should consider.

This section focuses on steps dementia patients (all adults) should address, including forming a care team and understanding various therapy.

While written for dementia patients, I recommend every adult fulfill these tasks before you turn thirty. Waiting is our enemy for these two duties. Be prepared!

The section includes:

1. A starter to-do list for any adult diagnosed with a fatal disease such as dementia.
2. A care team plan.

Chapter 12: Starter To-do List for Somebody and Family once Diagnosed with Dementia.

Dementia patients, loved ones, and family must address several matters early in the disease, including care, financial decisions, living quarters, Living Will, and Power of Attorney.

While you have full or most of your cognitive skills, take care of the listed priorities before diagnosis or when diagnosed. Please do not consider the items covered in this section a complete care list, but a start you tailor to your needs.

Fail to cross these items off the list while you maintain your facilities causes much regret for patients and loved ones.

Your life is your ship, and for now, you remain the captain. Plan how your ship faces the coming storm and, when you can no longer captain the ship yourself, have it already determined who takes over the helm.

Now remains your last best chance to have a substantial say in your future.

Care

Family, loved ones, and dementia patients must make difficult decisions concerning if somebody can become the primary volunteer caregiver. While dementia patients do not require 24/7 care in the early stage, it becomes necessary in the middle to late stages.

Nobody can get through dementia without others providing years of caregiving. While rare dementias kill in months, most dementia patients live for 5-20 years, with dementia growing progressively worse.

Diagnosed with dementia or in perfect health, we all must ask ourselves who would take care of us if dementia or another devastating disorder struck, requiring long-term caregiving.

Most families cannot afford professional caregiving, and the government will not help until towards the end, so family and loved ones must.

In an ideal world, we ask ourselves these tough questions and have a plan in place should something happen. This benefits not only those diagnosed with dementia but also the heroic voluntary caregivers who will see them to the end.

Financial Decisions

There are significant financial decisions to make, and earlier, the better.

Find out how much your insurance covers and the amount you must pay. A kinder world would not burden dementia patients, nor their loved ones, with overwhelming medical care costs.

In the United States and most countries in the world, the majority of dementia costs fall on families.

How Much Does Dementia Cost the Average Family?

With no urine or blood test for most dementia types, neurologists must rely on imaging and other expensive tests, often not to diagnose dementia but to rule out other neurological disorders.

Under the best scenario, related tests, doctor visits saddle the average patient with tens of thousands of dollars in deductibles by the time the neurological team diagnoses them with dementia. For some, such as dementia with Lewy bodies, it might run much higher as it can take up to eighteen months or longer before doctors make a correct diagnosis.

Our health system tells the average person: "Sorry, you have dementia. Oh, by the way, there's the bill."

Doctors, medical professionals, hospitals, drug companies, and others involved in treating dementia must make a living. Even when we factor out overcharging and profiteering, treating dementia would remain expensive.

The average American family's health insurance has deteriorated for years, the premiums growing too high, the deductibles unaffordable, and too many not worth the paper its written, much less the monthly premiums.

Authorities estimate the average cost per dementia patient is $341,840, with families expected to cover 70 percent.

Such a disease becomes a hardship for not only the patient but also their family. The demands, financial and otherwise, on voluntary caregivers often is devastating. Make difficult financial decisions early.

Financial costs vary from one dementia to another and the treatment plan.

Living Quarters

While most dementia patients maintain independence in stage one, at some point, they require help with daily tasks. Will somebody move in with her or him? Does the patient move in with somebody else? Will it become necessary for him or her to move into an assisted living community in later stages? If so, what type?

The person diagnosed should gather loved ones and decide such matters in the beginning. Like somebody on a small island with a hurricane approaching, one must be diligent. While no man or woman can withstand such a storm, they still take precautions to protect themselves and their families.

In part because of financial considerations, most families care for the loved one in the home until symptoms grow critical. Whether a dementia patient ends up in a special needs living facility is not a matter of if, but at what point for those who have access.

No matter how much love, care, and attention a voluntary caregiver or loved ones provide a dementia patient, they are ill-equipped to provide for somebody in the disorder's final stretch.

Families without access do the best they can to provide comfort for the loved one but make no mistake, the patient and family benefit if a special needs facility takes over at some point.

Which type of facility depends on which dementia and symptoms. Some dementias cause more cognitive problems, while others greater affect motor skills, some visual, and a few dementias cause more language problems. In the end, many dementias are more alike than not, as the damage to the brain spreads to other areas. Still, depending on the symptoms, different care facilities might be better than others.

Ask your neurologist or local dementia organizations about local facilities trained for your particular type. Hopefully, you live at home and maintain a normal or semi-normal life for years, but have a facility selected when the end grows near.

Living Will

Not to be confused with a Last Will and Testament that distributes assets, a living will focus on medical decisions. NOLO defines a living will.

> *A living will – sometimes called a health care declaration -- is a document in which you describe the kind of health care you want to receive if you are incapacitated and cannot speak for yourself. It is often paired with a power of attorney for health care, in which you name an agent to make health care decisions on your behalf. Some states combine these two documents into one document called an 'advanced directive.'*

It is crucial to document the dementia patient's wishes while you maintain facilities to make such decisions.

Use the Living Will to direct physicians to follow your wishes on what care you receive now and in the future when you might not maintain your cognitive skills.

Specify end-of-life medical treatment.

NOLO recommends prioritizing life-prolonging medical care, food, and water if you become unconscious, and palliative care, which we soon address[244].

Distribute copies of your living will to loved ones, doctors, insurance providers, and all health care facilities.

Power of Attorney

The American Bar Association describes a power of attorney:

> *A power of attorney gives one or more persons the power to act on your behalf as your agent. The power may be limited to a particular activity, such as closing the sale of your home or be general in its application. The power may give temporary or permanent authority to act on your behalf. The power may take effect immediately, or only upon the occurrence of a future event, usually a determination that you are unable to act for yourself due to mental or physical disability. The latter is called a "springing" power of attorney. A power of attorney may be revoked, but most states require written notice of revocation to the person named to act for you[245].*

It is important to establish a medical power of attorney to empower a trusted loved one to make medical decisions when a patient becomes incapable. If you do not choose the right person, you can almost count on the wrong people making important decisions down the road.

If you're in early stages dementia and reading this, you likely can still think clearly, but this changes as the symptoms worsen. The only way to protect a dementia patient's wishes when they lose their cognitive decision-making is by naming a power of attorney in advance.

Once you name a power of attorney, cover some dos and don'ts. After all, you are trusting another person with your life. Like with your doctors, speak your mind while you can and let people know what you expect.

As NOLO pointed out, some states merge the living will and power of attorney into an advanced directive. Whether together or separate, I recommend all adults, and particularly those diagnosed with dementia draw up a medical living will and name a power of attorney.

The starter to-do list provides a starting point for dementia patients, families, and any adult.

Once diagnosed, both the person diagnosed and loved ones must unite and build your to-do list. Add whatever makes sense for you and your unique situation.

Let's next cover a few key members of a dementia care team.

Chapter 13: CARE TEAM

The National Institute on Aging recommends building a care team.

The team includes an art therapist, mental health counselor, occupational therapist, palliative care specialist, physical therapist, and a speech therapist[246].

Art therapist

The art therapist reduces stress by engaging the patient in music and other expressive arts.

Since dementia causes enormous anxiety and mood swings, art therapists use music and art to soothe patients and assist caregivers. Most everybody responds to music. Some pump our blood and makes us want to shake our bodies to the rhythm. Other music helps us focus and achieve maximum concentration.

Some music geared towards dementia patients relaxes and calms. Music is a godsend!

Art is not a task but a love affair. Some say within each of us is an artist starving to escape. Art therapists use music and art as a brilliant tool to treat dementia anxiety, attention decline, sleep problems, etc.

Mental health counselors

A neurological disorder, dementia attacks the brain and inhibits cognitive skills. Mental health counselors help patients and families plan for the future and cope with the shock, hurt, and pain resulting from the diagnosis.

Most individuals and families suffer chronic mental stress when doctors diagnose a member with dementia.

Find a mental health counselor trained in dementia.

Turn to their expertise and do not allow the neurological disorder to destroy the remaining quality of life for the patient, or respond as a family in a way where dementia destroys many lives by one sweeping event.

Occupational therapists

The occupational therapist helps patients bathe, dress, eat, and perform daily tasks.

We think of the routine daily tasks as second nature, and it is as long as the neurons, pathways, arteries, heart, and brain perform as normal. When suffering a stroke or neurological disorder like dementia, we quickly learn nothing is second nature anymore. Like a child, dementia patients often must relearn how to perform basic tasks.

Occupational therapists help patients remain independent and then semi-independent, as long as possible, extending the quality of life. An occupational therapist is instrumental in treating most dementias.

Palliative care specialist

The palliative care specialist minimizes symptoms from diagnosis to the end. You or a loved one need somebody who addresses symptoms as soon as they arise, so find a quality palliative care specialist.

They extend the quality of life and reduce suffering.

Physical therapists

Physical therapists help motors skills by leading patients through exercise.

Although dementia is known as a mental disorder, what affects the brain affects the body and vice versa. Find a physical therapist trained to work with your specific dementia.

If you've seen somebody suffering Parkinsonism or other neurological disorders affecting movement, you have an idea of the problems some dementias cause, even in the earliest stages.

A physical therapist helps maintain balance and strength, allowing a person to walk and move on their own. As dementia progresses, so does the physical therapist's importance.

Speech therapists

The speech therapist addresses speech and swallowing problems, issues present in early dementia symptoms for some types, and eventually becomes a problem for most dementias.

What is the value of verbalizing one's thoughts, understanding what a loved one says, and swallowing our food without choking or causing infection by sending it down the wrong pipe?

These are issues speech therapists excel. The ones I've observed are passionate about helping people retrain the mind to overcome aphasia and swallowing problems.

Find a speech (and other types of) therapist trained in treating your specific type of dementia. These different listed therapists can minimize the long nightmare following a dementia diagnosis.

Chapter 14: LETTER TO CONGRESS

DEAR U.S. CONGRESS, NATIONS OF THE WORLD, & WEALTHY HUMANS

We call on the United States and the governments of the world to spend less on war and walls and more on Alzheimer's and dementia research.

If aliens were attacking us from another planet, I presume the nations of the world would unite against a common enemy. That is what I propose now.

The enemy I refer to does not come from another planet but threatens humans no less. Alzheimer's and dementia strike an American every 68 seconds and somebody worldwide every 30 seconds.

The nations of the world can save millions of lives and billions of dollars.

We need necessary funding to:

1. Discover the exact cause (s) of Alzheimer's and other dementias.
2. Develop accurate testing for Alzheimer's and other dementias.
3. Develop a vaccine to wipe out Alzheimer's and other dementias like we did polio.

Alzheimer's and dementia grow at a rate that will destroy the economies of most countries if we do not become more proactive.

We can save trillions of dollars for future generations if we invest now in discovering the exact cause (s), a vaccine to prevent it from happening, and other steps to defeat this horrifying disease.

Alzheimer's and other dementias threaten every family in all nations.

EARLY-ONSET ALZHEIMER'S DISEASE (EOAD)

We can do little for those with late-stage dementia, but the proposed steps might save millions of lives and trillions of dollars by diagnosing the different dementias early and treating them before they do significant damage.

Beller Health calls on politicians, corporations, and wealthy individuals to step forward to help win the war against dementia.

CONCLUSION

Thank you for reading this book. We covered a good amount of material.

Dementia is a cruel neurological disorder that robs people of their personalities, executive skills, memories, talents, language, voice, motor capabilities, and all that makes us individual humans.

Alzheimer's and Dementia

Although Alzheimer's disease (AD) is the most prevalent, we learned AD is to dementia what China is to Asia. Alzheimer's represents 60-80% of dementia, but 19 dementia types account for 99 percent.

Dementia Spares No Demographic

Dementia's reputation is known as an old folk's disease but strikes people all ages. Most dementia is not genetic, although certain types such as Huntington's disease are 100% familial.

Most Dementia is Incurable

Most dementia is incurable, but—if caught early enough—neurosurgeons can treat and sometimes reverse normal pressure hydrocephalus.

Dementia Prevalence

The first section focused on dementia as a general category. We learned 850,000 people in the UK have dementia, compared to 5.8 Americans and 50 million people worldwide.

Dementia Categories

We divided the 19 dementias into six categories:

- Lewy Body/Parkinsonism related dementias
- Alzheimer's related dementias
- Frontotemporal lobar degeneration related dementias
- Primary progressive aphasia related dementias
- Vascular dementias
- Other dementias

19 Dementia Types

Lewy Body/Parkinsonism Related Dementias

1. Dementia with Lewy Bodies
2. Parkinson's Disease Dementia
3. Corticobasal Syndrome

Alzheimer's Related Dementias

4. Typical Alzheimer's Disease
5. Posterior Cortical Atrophy
6. Down Syndrome with Alzheimer's
7. Limbic-predominant Age-related TDP-43 Encephalopathy (LATE)
8. Early-onset Alzheimer's

Frontotemporal Lobar Degeneration Related Dementias

9. Behavioral Variant Frontotemporal Dementia
10. Progressive Supranuclear Palsy

Primary Progressive Aphasia Related Dementias

11. Nonfluent Primary Progressive Aphasia (nfvPPA)

12. Logopenic Progressive Aphasia (LPA)

Vascular Dementia

13. *Cortical Vascular Dementia*
14. *Binswanger Disease*

Other Dementias

15. *Normal Pressure Hydrocephalus*
16. *Huntington's Disease*
17. *Korsakoff Syndrome*
18. *Creutzfeldt-Jakob Disease*
19. Amyotrophic Lateral Sclerosis

We examined the prevalence, costs, subtypes, symptoms, stages, and risk factors for early-onset Alzheimer's.

THE END

Of

EARLY-ONSET ALZHEIMER'S DISEASE (EOAD)

THANK YOU FOR READING

Thank you for reading the entire book. While this is not a literary work to enjoy, I hope you gained useful knowledge of dementia.

If you benefitted from this book, please take a moment to share your thoughts in a review. Reader reviews help other readers make educated decisions about this book before purchasing.

Book Review link for Early Onset Alzheimer's Disease (EOAD)

or

https://www.amazon.com/dp/B081R6D1R1

Look for annual updates to my health books, as I follow new studies and add any helpful information I find. Health and fitness are top priorities, and the heart and brain are my specialties.

I hope you develop the habits suggested in this book. Good luck on your health journey. Live long and prosper, my friend.

All the best,
Jerry Beller & Beller Health

BELLER HEALTH BOOKS

Beller Health Research Institute specializes in the heart and brain, and published the following Jerry Beller book series:
- Arrhythmia Series
- Vascular Disease Series
- 2020 Dementia Overview Series
- 19 Dementia Types Series

Please continue to view the books in each series.

Dementia Types, Symptoms, Stages, & Risk Factors Series

This book series is the first to cover each of the 19 primary dementia types.

20. _Dementia with Lewy Bodies_
21. _Parkinson's Disease Dementia_
22. _Corticobasal Syndrome_
23. _Typical Alzheimer's Disease_
24. _Posterior Cortical Atrophy_
25. _Down Syndrome with Alzheimer's_
26. _Limbic-predominant Age-related TDP-43 Encephalopathy (LATE)_
27. _Early-onset Alzheimer's_
28. _Behavioral Variant Frontotemporal Dementia_
29. _Progressive Supranuclear Palsy_
30. _Nonfluent Primary Progressive Aphasia_
31. _Logopenic Progressive Aphasia_
32. _Cortical Vascular Dementia_
33. _Binswanger Disease_
34. _Normal Pressure Hydrocephalus_
35. _Huntington's Disease_
36. _Korsakoff Syndrome_
37. _Creutzfeldt-Jakob Disease_
38. _Amyotrophic Lateral Sclerosis_

2020 Dementia Overview Series

Whereas in the *Dementia Types, Symptoms, Stages, and Risk Factors* series, each book covers a different dementia type, this series focuses on groups of dementias.

1. Dementia Types, Symptoms, & Stages
2. *Lewy Body/Parkinsonism Dementias*
3. *Vascular Dementia*
4. *Frontotemporal Dementia (FTD)*
5. Alzheimer's Related Dementias
6. *Prevent or Slow Dementia*

JERRY BELLER HEALTH RESEARCH INSTITUTE

Other Beller Health Books

You can view or purchase all Beller Health Books on Amazon at the following web address:

https://amzn.to/2TpDr8e

ABOUT THE AUTHOR

Jerry Beller is the lead author and researcher at Beller Medical Research Institute. Beller distinguished himself three times in the medical world by being the first to write and publish books on particular dementia fields.

He wrote the first book covering all 15 primary dementia types, which he since expanded to cover nineteen. Beller followed this accomplishment by writing a book on each dementia type. He broke medical ground a third time when he published the first book on the new dementia category LATE.

When the world struggled to grasp the difference between Alzheimer's disease and China, Beller explained:

> *Alzheimer's is only one dementia, much like China is only one country in Asia. Just as we do not want to ignore the other countries in Asia because China is the largest, nor do we want to ignore the less prevalent dementia types.*

Despite his accomplishments, he remains humble. "Until we win the dementia war, I've no reason to celebrate," Beller said. "If we win the war during my lifetime, I will celebrate with a few hundred brothers and sisters around the world who share my passion. Until then, we have too much work left to worry about accolades and legacies."

When not researching dementia, Jerry enjoys life with his wife of thirty-plus years, Nicola, and their two children.

Visit Jerry Beller:

https://bellerhealth.com

1 'What Is Dementia?', *Alzheimer's Disease and Dementia* <https://alz.org/alzheimers-dementia/what-is-dementia> [accessed 18 September 2019].

2 'What Is Dementia? Symptoms, Types, and Diagnosis', *National Institute on Aging* <https://www.nia.nih.gov/health/what-dementia-symptoms-types-and-diagnosis> [accessed 18 September 2019].

[3] 'What Is Dementia?', *Alzheimer's Society* <https://www.alzheimers.org.uk/about-dementia/types-dementia/what-dementia> [accessed 18 September 2019].

[4] 'Dementia' <https://www.who.int/news-room/fact-sheets/detail/dementia> [accessed 18 September 2019].

[5] 'Risk Factors' <https://stanfordhealthcare.org/medical-conditions/brain-and-nerves/dementia/risk-factors.html> [accessed 20 September 2019].

[6] W. M. van der Flier and P. Scheltens, 'Epidemiology and Risk Factors of Dementia', *Journal of Neurology, Neurosurgery & Psychiatry*, 76.suppl 5 (2005), v2–7 <https://doi.org/10.1136/jnnp.2005.082867>.

[7] Kent Allen, 'Dementia Rates to Grow for African Americans, Hispanics', *AARP* <http://www.aarp.org/health/dementia/info-2018/dementia-alzheimer-cases-grow-nonwhites.html> [accessed 20 September 2019].

[8] Elizabeth Rose Mayeda and others, 'Inequalities in Dementia Incidence between Six Racial and Ethnic Groups over 14 Years', *Alzheimer's & Dementia: The Journal of the Alzheimer's Association*, 12.3 (2016), 216–24 <https://doi.org/10.1016/j.jalz.2015.12.007>.

[9] 'African Americans at Higher Dementia Risk than Other Racial Groups', *Reuters*, 10 March 2016 <https://www.reuters.com/article/us-health-dementia-race-u-s-idUSKCN0WC2X5> [accessed 20 September 2019].

[10] Steve Ford, 'Likelihood of Dementia "Higher among Black Ethnic Groups"', *Nursing Times*, 2018 <https://www.nursingtimes.net/news/research-and-innovation/likelihood-of-dementia-higher-among-black-ethnic-groups-08-08-2018/> [accessed 21 September 2019].

[11] 'Dementia' <https://www.who.int/news-room/fact-sheets/detail/dementia> [accessed 21 September 2019].

[12] 'Women and Alzheimer's', *Alzheimer's Disease and Dementia* <https://alz.org/alzheimers-dementia/what-is-alzheimers/women-and-alzheimer-s> [accessed 21 September 2019].

[13] 'Dementia Facts', *Dementia Consortium* <https://www.dementiaconsortium.org/dementia-facts/> [accessed 21 September 2019].

[14] 'Dementia' <https://www.who.int/news-room/fact-sheets/detail/dementia> [accessed 21 September 2019].

[15] 'Why Is Dementia Different for Women?', *Alzheimer's Society* <https://www.alzheimers.org.uk/blog/why-dementia-different-women> [accessed 21 September 2019].

[16] Jessica L. Podcasy and C. Neill Epperson, 'Considering Sex and Gender in Alzheimer Disease and Other Dementias', *Dialogues in Clinical Neuroscience*, 18.4 (2016), 437–46 <https://www.ncbi.nlm.nih.gov/pmc/articles/PMC5286729/> [accessed 21 September 2019].

[17] 'WHO | Life Expectancy', *WHO* <http://www.who.int/gho/mortality_burden_disease/life_tables/situation_trends_text/en/> [accessed 21 September 2019].

[18] 'Products - Data Briefs - Number 328 - November 2018', 2019 <https://www.cdc.gov/nchs/products/databriefs/db328.htm> [accessed 21 September 2019].

[19] Jacqui Thornton, 'WHO Report Shows That Women Outlive Men Worldwide', *BMJ*, 365 (2019), l1631 <https://doi.org/10.1136/bmj.l1631>.

[20] 'Why Do Women Live Longer Than Men?', *Time* <https://time.com/5538099/why-do-women-live-longer-than-men/> [accessed 21 September 2019].

[21] 'Dementia' <https://www.who.int/news-room/fact-sheets/detail/dementia> [accessed 20 September 2019].

[22] 'Alzheimer's Disease: Facts & Figures', *BrightFocus Foundation*, 2015 <https://www.brightfocus.org/alzheimers/article/alzheimers-disease-facts-figures> [accessed 4 September 2019].

[23] 'Facts for the Media', *Alzheimer's Society* <https://www.alzheimers.org.uk/about-us/news-and-media/facts-media> [accessed 20 September 2019].

[24] 'Countries With The Highest Rates Of Deaths From Dementia',

WorldAtlas <https://www.worldatlas.com/articles/countries-with-the-highest-rates-of-deaths-from-dementia.html> [accessed 20 September 2019].

[25] 'World Alzheimer Report 2018 - The State of the Art of Dementia Research: New Frontiers', *NEW FRONTIERS*, 48.

[26] 'ALZHEIMERS/DEMENTIA DEATH RATE BY COUNTRY', *World Life Expectancy* <https://www.worldlifeexpectancy.com/cause-of-death/alzheimers-dementia/by-country/> [accessed 24 September 2019].

[27] 'Alzheimer Europe - Research - European Collaboration on Dementia - Cost of Dementia - Regional/National Cost of Illness Estimates' <https://www.alzheimer-europe.org/Research/European-Collaboration-on-Dementia/Cost-of-dementia/Regional-National-cost-of-illness-estimates> [accessed 26 September 2019].

[28] 'Publications | NATSEM' <https://www.natsem.canberra.edu.au/publications/?publication=economic-cost-of-dementia-in-australia-2016-2056> [accessed 22 September 2019].

[29] 'Dementia UK Report', *Alzheimer's Society* <https://www.alzheimers.org.uk/about-us/policy-and-influencing/dementia-uk-report> [accessed 22 September 2019].

[30] 'Dementia Statistics – U.S. & Worldwide Stats', *BrainTest*, 2015 <https://braintest.com/dementia-stats-u-s-worldwide/> [accessed 23 September 2019].

[31] 'Newsroom | Northwestern Mutual - 2018 C.A.R.E. Study', *Newsroom | Northwestern Mutual* <https://news.northwesternmutual.com/2018-care-study> [accessed 22 September 2019].

[32] 'ALZHEIMERS/DEMENTIA DEATH RATE BY COUNTRY'.

[33] 'Alzheimer Europe - Research - European Collaboration on Dementia - Cost of Dementia - Regional/National Cost of Illness Estimates'.

[34] 'Publications | NATSEM'.

[35] 'Dementia UK Report'.

[36] 'Dementia Statistics – U.S. & Worldwide Stats'.

[37] 'What Is Alzheimer's Disease?', *National Institute on Aging* <https://www.nia.nih.gov/health/what-alzheimers-disease> [accessed 28 November 2018].

[38] '2017-Facts-and-Figures.Pdf'

<https://www.alz.org/documents_custom/2017-facts-and-figures.pdf> [accessed 18 February 2018].

[39] 'Alzheimer's Society of America□» Alzheimer's Disease' <http://alzheimerssocietyofamerica.org/dementia/alzheimers-disease/> [accessed 18 February 2018].

[40] 'What Is Alzheimer's?', *Alzheimer's Disease and Dementia* <https://alz.org/alzheimers-dementia/what-is-alzheimers> [accessed 28 November 2018].

[41] 'Alzheimer's Disease - Symptoms and Causes', *Mayo Clinic* <http://www.mayoclinic.org/diseases-conditions/alzheimers-disease/symptoms-causes/syc-20350447> [accessed 29 November 2018].

[42] 'Alzheimer's Disease', *Alzheimer's Society* <https://www.alzheimers.org.uk/about-dementia/types-dementia/alzheimers-disease> [accessed 28 November 2018].

[43] <img src='//sgec stanford edu/content/dam/sm-profiles/profileBGoldmanM jpg img 620 high png' alt='Bruce Goldman'> By Bruce Goldman Bruce Goldman is a science writer for the medical school's Office of Communication & Public Affairs, 'Scientists Reveal How Beta-Amyloid May Cause Alzheimer's', *News Center* <http://med.stanford.edu/news/all-news/2013/09/scientists-reveal-how-beta-amyloid-may-cause-alzheimers.html> [accessed 12 December 2018].

[44] 'What Is Alzheimer's Disease?', *National Institute on Aging* <https://www.nia.nih.gov/health/what-alzheimers-disease> [accessed 12 December 2018].

[45] Robin Seaton Jefferson, 'UT Southwestern Medical Center Researchers Discover Alzheimer's Vaccine, Hope To Test In Humans Soon', *Forbes* <https://www.forbes.com/sites/robinseatonjefferson/2018/11/23/ut-researchers-discover-alzheimers-vaccine-hope-to-test-in-humans-soon/> [accessed 12 December 2018].

[46] Roger N. Rosenberg, Min Fu, and Doris Lambracht-Washington, 'Active Full-Length DNA Aβ42 Immunization in 3xTg-AD Mice Reduces Not Only Amyloid Deposition but Also Tau Pathology', *Alzheimer's Research & Therapy*, 10.1 (2018), 115 <https://doi.org/10.1186/s13195-018-0441-4>.

[47] 'Symptoms of Early Onset Dementia' <https://www.hopkinsmedicine.org/healthlibrary/conditions/adult/nervous_system_disorders/early-onset_alzheimer_disease_134,63> [accessed 29

November 2018].

[48] 'Younger/Early Onset', *Alzheimer's Disease and Dementia* <https://alz.org/alzheimers-dementia/what-is-alzheimers/younger-early-onset> [accessed 12 December 2018].

[49] 'Symptoms of Early Onset Dementia' <https://www.hopkinsmedicine.org/healthlibrary/conditions/adult/nervous_system_disorders/early-onset_alzheimer_disease_134,63> [accessed 12 December 2018].

[50] The Editors, 'What Is Alzheimer's Disease? A Visual Primer', *Scientific American* <https://www.scientificamerican.com/article/what-is-alzheimers-disease-visual-primer/> [accessed 13 December 2018].

[51] 'Number of Alzheimer's Deaths Found to Be Underreported', *National Institute on Aging* <https://www.nia.nih.gov/news/number-alzheimers-deaths-found-be-underreported> [accessed 13 December 2018].

[52] 'Prevalence of Alzheimer's', 1.

[53] '2018 Alzheimer's Disease Facts and Figures', *Alzheimer's & Dementia: The Journal of the Alzheimer's Association*, 14.3 (2018), 367–429 <https://doi.org/10.1016/j.jalz.2018.02.001>.

[54] CDC, 'Deaths from Alzheimer's Disease', *Centers for Disease Control and Prevention*, 2017 <https://www.cdc.gov/features/alzheimers-disease-deaths/index.html> [accessed 13 December 2018].

[55] 'Alzheimer's Disease: Facts & Figures', *BrightFocus Foundation*, 2015 <https://www.brightfocus.org/alzheimers/article/alzheimers-disease-facts-figures> [accessed 30 November 2018].

[56] 'Latest Estimate: One New Case of Dementia Every 3.2 Seconds Archives', *Dementia Alliance International* <https://www.dementiaallianceinternational.org/tag/latest-estimate-one-new-case-of-dementia-every-3-2-seconds/> [accessed 13 December 2018].

[57] 'Dementia' <https://www.who.int/news-room/fact-sheets/detail/dementia> [accessed 13 December 2018].

[58] 'World Alzheimer Report 2018 - The State of the Art of Dementia Research: New Frontiers', *NEW FRONTIERS*, 48.

[59] 'Causes of Death', *Our World in Data* <https://ourworldindata.org/causes-of-death> [accessed 13 December 2018].

[60] 'Dementia Risk Factors', *Queensland Brain Institute*, 2017 <https://qbi.uq.edu.au/dementia/dementia-risk-factors> [accessed 13

December 2018].

[61] 'How Does Alzheimer's Affect Women and Men Differently? | Cognitive Vitality | Alzheimer's Drug Discovery Foundation' <https://www.alzdiscovery.org/cognitive-vitality/blog/how-does-alzheimers-affect-women-and-men-differently> [accessed 13 December 2018].

[62] E Willetta St, 'As Our Country Ages, the Number of People Touched by Alzheimer's Only Continues to Increase. Already, More than a Third of the U.S. Adult Population Has Some Personal Connection to the Disease, through a Spouse, Family Member or Other Blood Relative.', 2.

[63] 'How Alzheimer's Could Be Type 2 Diabetes', *Alzheimers.Net*, 2016 <https://www.alzheimers.net/2015-10-14/how-alzheimers-could-be-type-2-diabetes/> [accessed 13 December 2018].

[64] 'Facts about the Connection between Down Syndrome and Alzheimer's Disease', *Global Down Syndrome Foundation*, 2012 <https://www.globaldownsyndrome.org/about-down-syndrome/facts-about-down-syndrome/facts-about-the-connection-between-down-syndrome-and-alzheimers-disease/> [accessed 13 December 2018].

[65] 'Higher Blood Pressure at Midlife Increases Your Risk for Dementia' <https://www.alzheimers.net/higher-blood-pressure-increases-your-risk-for-dementia/> [accessed 13 December 2018].

[66] J. Carson Smith and others, 'Physical Activity and Brain Function in Older Adults at Increased Risk for Alzheimer's Disease', *Brain Sciences*, 3.1 (2013), 54–83 <https://doi.org/10.3390/brainsci3010054>.

[67] 'Obesity: A Risk Factor for Alzheimer's', *Health Essentials from Cleveland Clinic*, 2013 <https://health.clevelandclinic.org/obesity-a-risk-factor-for-alzheimers/> [accessed 13 December 2018].

[68] 'Nine Lifestyle Factors May Lower Your Alzheimer's Risk | Cognitive Vitality | Alzheimer's Drug Discovery Foundation' <https://www.alzdiscovery.org/cognitive-vitality/blog/nine-lifestyle-factors-may-lower-your-alzheimers-risk> [accessed 13 December 2018].

[69] 'Geoba.Se: Gazetteer - United States - 2019 - Statistics and Rankings' <http://www.geoba.se/country.php?cc=US&year=2019> [accessed 28 November 2018].

[70] Adrian O'Dowd, 'Dementia Is Now Leading Cause of Death in Women in England', *BMJ*, 358 (2017), j3445 <https://doi.org/10.1136/bmj.j3445>.

[71] 'Deaths Registered in England and Wales (Series DR) - Office for

National Statistics' <https://www.ons.gov.uk/peoplepopulationandcommunity/birthsdeathsandmarriages/deaths/bulletins/deathsregisteredinenglandandwalesseriesdr/2016> [accessed 13 December 2018].

[72] 'Women and Alzheimer's Disease: A Global Epidemic', *NWHN*, 2015 <https://www.nwhn.org/women-and-alzheimers-disease-a-global-epidemic/> [accessed 13 December 2018].

[73] 'WHO | Top 10 Causes of Death', *WHO* <https://doi.org//entity/gho/mortality_burden_disease/causes_death/top_10/en/index.html>.

[74] Yan Zhou and others, 'African Americans Are Less Likely to Enroll in Preclinical Alzheimer's Disease Clinical Trials', *Alzheimer's & Dementia: Translational Research & Clinical Interventions*, 3.1 (2017), 57–64 <https://doi.org/10.1016/j.trci.2016.09.004>.

[75] 'Likelihood of Dementia Higher among Black Ethnic Groups', *EurekAlert!* <https://www.eurekalert.org/pub_releases/2018-08/ucl-lod080618.php> [accessed 13 December 2018].

[76] 'Likelihood of Dementia Higher among Black Ethnic Groups' <https://medicalxpress.com/news/2018-08-likelihood-dementia-higher-black-ethnic.html> [accessed 13 December 2018].

[77] 'Dementia Rates Higher among Black People, New Study Finds', *The Independent*, 2018 <https://www.independent.co.uk/news/health/dementia-black-white-asian-ethnicity-alzheimers-disease-memory-a8481786.html> [accessed 13 December 2018].

[78] 'New Alzheimer's Association Report Reveals Sharp Increases in Alzheimer's Prevalence, Deaths and Cos', *Alzheimer's Disease and Dementia* <https://alz.org/news/2018/new_alzheimer_s_association_report_reveals_sharp_i> [accessed 13 December 2018].

[79] Liesi E. Hebert and others, 'Alzheimer Disease in the United States (2010–2050) Estimated Using the 2010 Census', *Neurology*, 80.19 (2013), 1778–83 <https://doi.org/10.1212/WNL.0b013e31828726f5>.

[80] 'The 50 US States Ranked By Population', *WorldAtlas* <https://www.worldatlas.com/articles/us-states-by-population.html> [accessed 30 November 2018].

[81] 'Dementia Statistics – U.S. & Worldwide Stats', *BrainTest*, 2015 <https://braintest.com/dementia-stats-u-s-worldwide/> [accessed 1 December 2018].

[82] 'Americans With Alzheimer's Now Number 5.7 Million' <https://www.forbes.com/sites/nextavenue/2018/03/25/americans-with-alzheimers-now-number-5-7-million/#70db8124b627> [accessed 1 December 2018].

[83] 'Fiscal Year 2019 Alzheimer's Research Funding', 1.

[84] 'Alzheimer's Disease'.

[85] 'Facts and Figures', *Alzheimer's Disease and Dementia* <https://alz.org/alzheimers-dementia/facts-figures> [accessed 30 November 2018].

[86] Bruce Japsen, 'Alzheimer's Costs Reach $277 Billion', *Forbes* <https://www.forbes.com/sites/brucejapsen/2018/03/20/alzheimers-costs-reach-277-billion/> [accessed 29 November 2018].

[87] 'WHO | Dementia Cases Set to Triple by 2050 but Still Largely Ignored', *WHO* <https://www.who.int/mediacentre/news/releases/2012/dementia_20120411/en/> [accessed 30 November 2018].

[88] 'Ten Countries with the Highest Population in the World' <https://www.internetworldstats.com/stats8.htm> [accessed 30 November 2018].

[89] 'How Many Countries Are There in the World? (2018) - Total & List | Worldometers' <http://www.worldometers.info/geography/how-many-countries-are-there-in-the-world/> [accessed 30 November 2018].

[90] Jianping Jia and others, 'The Cost of Alzheimer's Disease in China and Re-Estimation of Costs Worldwide', *Alzheimer's & Dementia: The Journal of the Alzheimer's Association*, 14.4 (2018), 483–91 <https://doi.org/10.1016/j.jalz.2017.12.006>.

[91] '2018 Alzheimer's Facts & Figures' <http://www.alzheimersweekly.com/2018/03/2018-alzheimers-facts-figures.html> [accessed 13 December 2018].

[92] 'Alzheimer's Disease Consists of Three Distinct Subtypes, According to UCLA Study', *UCLA* <http://newsroom.ucla.edu/releases/alzheimers-disease-consists-of-three-distinct-subtypes-according-to-ucla-study> [accessed 12 November 2019].

[93] 'When Alzheimer's Symptoms Start before Age 65', *Mayo Clinic* <https://www.mayoclinic.org/diseases-conditions/alzheimers-disease/in-depth/alzheimers/art-20048356> [accessed 2 December 2019].

[94] Genetics Home Reference, 'What Is a Chromosome?', *Genetics*

Home Reference <https://ghr.nlm.nih.gov/primer/basics/chromosome> [accessed 2 December 2019].

[95] 'What Are Chromosomes?' <https://www.healio.com/hematology-oncology/learn-genomics/genomics-primer/what-are-chromosomes> [accessed 2 December 2019].

[96] File:Chromosome-es svg: KES47, *English: Graphic Decomposition of a Chromosome (Found in the Cell Nucleus), to the Bases Pair of the DNA.*, 2010, File:Chromosome-es.svg <https://commons.wikimedia.org/wiki/File:Chromosome_en.svg> [accessed 2 December 2019].

[97] Genetics Home Reference, 'Chromosome 1', *Genetics Home Reference* <https://ghr.nlm.nih.gov/chromosome/1> [accessed 2 December 2019].

[98] Genetics Home Reference, 'PSEN2 Gene', *Genetics Home Reference* <https://ghr.nlm.nih.gov/gene/PSEN2> [accessed 2 December 2019].

[99] 'Chromosome 21 - an Overview | ScienceDirect Topics' <https://www.sciencedirect.com/topics/neuroscience/chromosome-21> [accessed 3 December 2019].

[100] National Human Genome Research Institute, *English: Human Male Karyotype after G-Banding. Chromosome 21 Highlighted*, 2015, File:Human male karyotype high resolution.jpg <https://commons.wikimedia.org/wiki/File:Human_male_karyotype_high_resolution_-_Chromosome_21.png> [accessed 1 December 2019].

[101] Thomas D. Bird, 'Early-Onset Familial Alzheimer Disease', in *GeneReviews®*, ed. by Margaret P. Adam and others (Seattle (WA): University of Washington, Seattle, 1993) <http://www.ncbi.nlm.nih.gov/books/NBK1236/> [accessed 25 December 2019].

[102] 'Alzheimer's Disease Type 3 (AD3)', *Centogene*, 2018 <https://www.centogene.com/science/centopedia/alzheimers-disease-type-3-ad3.html> [accessed 25 December 2019].

[103] 'Alzheimer Disease 3' <https://www.uniprot.org/diseases/DI-00086> [accessed 25 December 2019].

[104] **Byron Creese and others, 'AN EVALUATION OF PREDICTORS AND COGNITIVE DECLINE ASSOCIATED WITH PERSISTENT AND TRANSIENT PSYCHOTIC**

SYMPTOMS IN ALZHEIMER'S DISEASE', *Alzheimer's & Dementia: The Journal of the Alzheimer's Association*, 13.7 (2017), P367 <https://doi.org/10.1016/j.jalz.2017.06.315>.

[105] Ilona Hallikainen and others, 'The Progression of Neuropsychiatric Symptoms in Alzheimer's Disease During a Five-Year Follow-Up: Kuopio ALSOVA Study', *Journal of Alzheimer's Disease*, 61.4 (2018), 1367–76 <https://doi.org/10.3233/JAD-170697>.

[106] Sheridan T. Read, Christine Toye, and Dianne Wynaden, 'Experiences and Expectations of Living with Dementia: A Qualitative Study', *Collegian*, 24.5 (2017), 427–32 <https://doi.org/10.1016/j.colegn.2016.09.003>.

[107] undefined, 'How to Tell Alzheimer's Disease from "normal" Memory Loss', *Cleveland.Com*, 2011 <http://www.cleveland.com/healthfit/index.ssf/2011/04/how_to_tell_alzheimers_disease.html> [accessed 14 December 2018].

[108] 'When a Person with Alzheimer's Rummages and Hides Things', *National Institute on Aging* <https://www.nia.nih.gov/health/when-person-alzheimers-rummages-and-hides-things> [accessed 14 December 2018].

[109] Katherine Kam, 'Memory Loss With Alzheimer's Disease: What to Expect', *WebMD* <https://www.webmd.com/alzheimers/features/dealing-with-alzheimers-disease-memory-loss> [accessed 14 December 2018].

[110] Tara E. Tracy and Li Gan, 'Acetylated Tau in Alzheimer's Disease: An Instigator of Synaptic Dysfunction Underlying Memory Loss', *BioEssays*, 39.4 (2017), n/a-n/a <https://doi.org/10.1002/bies.201600224>.

[111] 'Brain Tour', *Alzheimer's Disease and Dementia* <https://alz.org/alzheimers-dementia/what-is-alzheimers/brain_tour> [accessed 14 December 2018].

[112] Holger Jahn, 'Memory Loss in Alzheimer's Disease', *Dialogues in Clinical Neuroscience*, 15.4 (2013), 445–54 <https://www.ncbi.nlm.nih.gov/pmc/articles/PMC3898682/> [accessed 14 December 2018].

[113] 'How Do People Experience Memory Loss?', *Alzheimer's Society* <https://www.alzheimers.org.uk/about-dementia/symptoms-and-diagnosis/symptoms/memory-loss-in-dementia> [accessed 14 December 2018].

[114] 'Memory Loss: When to Seek Help', *Mayo Clinic* <https://www.mayoclinic.org/diseases-conditions/alzheimers-disease/in-depth/memory-loss/art-20046326> [accessed 14 December 2018].

[115] 'Normal Aging vs Dementia | Alzheimer Society of Canada' <http://alzheimer.ca/en/Home/About-dementia/What-is-dementia/Normal-aging-vs-dementia> [accessed 14 December 2018].

[116] 'Alzheimer's Disease', *Memory and Aging Center* <https://memory.ucsf.edu/alzheimer-disease> [accessed 14 December 2018].

[117] Nancy L. Mace and Peter V. Rabins, *The 36-Hour Day: A Family Guide to Caring for People Who Have Alzheimer Disease, Other Dementias, and Memory Loss* (JHU Press, 2017).

[118] 'When Alzheimer's Turns Violent' <http://www.cnn.com/2011/HEALTH/03/30/alzheimers.violence.caregiving/index.html> [accessed 14 December 2018].

[119] 'Alzheimer's: 25 Signs Never to Ignore' <https://www.cbsnews.com/pictures/alzheimers-25-signs-never-to-ignore/> [accessed 14 December 2018].

[120] 'Treatments for Behavior', *Alzheimer's Disease and Dementia* <https://alz.org/alzheimers-

dementia/treatments/treatments-for-behavior> [accessed 14 December 2018].

[121] 'What Causes Aggressive Behaviour?', *Alzheimer's Society* <https://www.alzheimers.org.uk/about-dementia/symptoms-and-diagnosis/symptoms/what-causes-aggression-dementia> [accessed 14 December 2018].

[122] 'Five Tips for Safely Managing Aggressive Behavior in Someone with Alzheimer's', *BrightFocus Foundation*, 2016 <https://www.brightfocus.org/alzheimers/article/five-tips-safely-managing-aggressive-behavior-someone-alzheimers> [accessed 14 December 2018].

[123] 'Coping with Agitation and Aggression in Alzheimer's Disease', *National Institute on Aging* <https://www.nia.nih.gov/health/coping-agitation-and-aggression-alzheimers-disease> [accessed 14 December 2018].

[124] Nancy J. Donovan and others, 'Longitudinal Association of Amyloid Beta and Anxious-Depressive Symptoms in Cognitively Normal Older Adults', *American Journal of Psychiatry*, 175.6 (2018), 530–37 <https://doi.org/10.1176/appi.ajp.2017.17040442>.

[125] 'Anxiety Disorders Could Lead to Alzheimer's', *Alzheimers.Net*, 2018 <https://www.alzheimers.net/anxiety-disorders-could-lead-to-alzheimers/> [accessed 14 December 2018].

[126] Noora-Maria Suhonen and others, 'The Modified Frontal Behavioral Inventory (FBI-Mod) for Patients with Frontotemporal Lobar Degeneration, Alzheimer's Disease, and Mild Cognitive Impairment', *Journal of Alzheimer's Disease*, 56.4 (2017), 1241–51 <https://doi.org/10.3233/JAD-160983>.

[127] Farrah Daly and others, '"Neither Gone nor Here": Coping with Personality Change and Loss of Identity in

Neurologic Disease (FR415)', *Journal of Pain and Symptom Management*, 55.2 (2018), 601–2 <https://doi.org/10.1016/j.jpainsymman.2017.12.096>.

[128] 'The Physical Symptoms of Alzheimer's | ASC Blog', *Senior Living Communities & Nursing Homes in Indiana | ASC*, 2015 <https://www.asccare.com/the-physical-symptoms-of-alzheimers/> [accessed 15 December 2018].

[129] 'Alzheimer's Disease - Causes, Symptoms, Prevention - Southern Cross NZ' <https://www.southerncross.co.nz/group/medical-library/alzheimers-disease-causes-symptoms-prevention> [accessed 15 December 2018].

[130] Hillary Hollman, 'Recognizing The Physical Signs Of Alzheimer's Disease', *AIHC*, 2015 <https://www.americaninhomecare.com/blog/2015/08/27/physical-signs-of-alzheimers-disease/> [accessed 15 December 2018].

[131] 'Alzheimer's Disease - Symptoms and Causes', *Mayo Clinic* <https://www.mayoclinic.org/diseases-conditions/alzheimers-disease/symptoms-causes/syc-20350447> [accessed 15 December 2018].

[132] 'Alzheimer's Disease Complications: Physical and Mental', *Healthline*, 2014 <https://www.healthline.com/health/alzheimers-disease-complications> [accessed 15 December 2018].

[133] Alexandra J. Mably and others, 'Impairments in Spatial Representations and Rhythmic Coordination of Place Cells in the 3xTg Mouse Model of Alzheimer's Disease', *Hippocampus*, 27.4 (2017), 378–92 <https://doi.org/10.1002/hipo.22697>.

[134] Eleonora M. Lad and others, 'Evaluation of Inner Retinal Layers as Biomarkers in Mild Cognitive Impairment to Moderate Alzheimer's Disease', *PLOS ONE*, 13.2 (2018),

e0192646 <https://doi.org/10.1371/journal.pone.0192646>.

[135] Richard F. Uhlmann and others, 'Visual Impairment and Cognitive Dysfunction in Alzheimer's Disease', *Journal of General Internal Medicine*, 6.2 (1991), 126–32 <https://doi.org/10.1007/BF02598307>.

[136] 'How Alzheimer's Disease Affects Vision and Perception - VisionAware' <http://www.visionaware.org/info/for-seniors/health-and-aging/vision-loss-and-the-challenges-of-aging/alzheimer%27s-disease/how-alzheimer%E2%80%99s-disease-affects-vision-and-perception/12345> [accessed 15 December 2018].

[137] 'Posterior Cortical Atrophy', *Memory and Aging Center* <https://memory.ucsf.edu/posterior-cortical-atrophy> [accessed 15 December 2018].

[138] Claudia Metzler-Baddeley and others, 'Visual Impairment in Posterior Cortical Atrophy and Dementia with Lewy Bodies', *Alzheimer's & Dementia: The Journal of the Alzheimer's Association*, 5.4 (2009), P458 <https://doi.org/10.1016/j.jalz.2009.04.862>.

[139] 'Supporting People with Sight Loss and Dementia', *RNIB - See Differently*, 2014 <https://www.rnib.org.uk/services-we-offer-advice-professionals-nb-magazine-health-professionals-nb-features/supporting> [accessed 15 December 2018].

[140] 'Alzheimer's Disease - American Foundation for the Blind' <http://www.afb.org/section.aspx?SectionID=63&TopicID=291&DocumentID=3213&rewrite=0> [accessed 15 December 2018].

[141] 'Sight Loss - Dementia and Sensory Loss - SCIE' <https://www.scie.org.uk/dementia/living-with-dementia/sensory-loss/sight-loss.asp> [accessed 15

December 2018].

[142] 'Sight, Perception and Hallucinations in Dementia', 14.

[143] Fernando Cuetos and others, 'Word Recognition in Alzheimer's Disease: Effects of Semantic Degeneration', *Journal of Neuropsychology*, 11.1 (2017), 26–39 <https://doi.org/10.1111/jnp.12077>.

[144] 'Symptoms & Causes: Mesulam Center for Cognitive Neurology and Alzheimer's Disease: Feinberg School of Medicine: Northwestern University' <https://www.brain.northwestern.edu/dementia/ppa/signs.html> [accessed 15 December 2018].

[145] 'Stages of Alzheimer's Disease | Johns Hopkins Medicine Health Library' <https://www.hopkinsmedicine.org/healthlibrary/conditions/nervous_system_disorders/stages_of_alzheimers_disease_134,64> [accessed 18 December 2018].

[146] 'One-Third of Seniors Die With Alzheimer's Disease', *Health Essentials from Cleveland Clinic*, 2013 <https://health.clevelandclinic.org/one-third-of-seniors-die-with-alzheimers-disease/> [accessed 18 December 2018].

[147] CDC, 'Disease of the Week - Alzheimer's Disease', *Centers for Disease Control and Prevention*, 2018 <http://www.cdc.gov/dotw/alzheimers/index.html> [accessed 18 December 2018].

[148] 'World Alzheimer's Day – Global Alzheimer's & Dementia Action Alliance (GADAA)' <https://www.gadaalliance.org/news/take-action-for-world-alzheimers-day/> [accessed 18 December 2018].

[149] 'World Alzheimer Report 2018 - The State of the Art of Dementia Research: New Frontiers', *NEW FRONTIERS*, 48.

150 'Stages of Alzheimer's Disease: Progression and Outlook', *Medical News Today* <https://www.medicalnewstoday.com/articles/315123.php> [accessed 19 December 2018].

151 'What Are the 7 Stages of Alzheimer's Disease?', *Alzheimers.Net* <https://www.alzheimers.net/stages-of-alzheimers-disease/> [accessed 19 December 2018].

152 'The Stages of Alzheimer's Disease' <https://www.agingcare.com/articles/stages-of-alzheimers-disease-118964.htm> [accessed 19 December 2018].

153 'What Are the 7 Stages of Alzheimer's Disease? Symptoms & Signs', *MedicineNet* <https://www.medicinenet.com/alzheimers_disease_symptoms_and_stages/article.htm> [accessed 19 December 2018].

154 'Alzheimer's: Recognising the Stages' <https://www.elder.org/dementia-care/alzheimers-recognising-the-stages/> [accessed 19 December 2018].

155 'Stages & Progression', *Alzheimer Society of Ireland* <https://www.alzheimer.ie/About-Dementia/Stages-progression.aspx> [accessed 19 December 2018].

156 'Stages of Alzheimer's Disease' <https://www.arc-ct.org/stages_of_alzheimers_disease.php> [accessed 19 December 2018].

157 'The Seven Stages of Alzheimer's | Brain Matters Research' <http://brainmattersresearch.com/the-seven-stages-of-alzheimers/> [accessed 19 December 2018].

158 'Hospice and the Alzheimer's Patient: What You Need to Know', *Pathways Home Health and Hospice* <https://www.pathwayshealth.org/hospice-topics/hospice-alzheimer%c2%80%c2%99s-patient-need-know/> [accessed 19 December 2018].

159 'WBHI Think Tank | 7 Stages of Alzheimer's – 7

Levels of Dementia' <https://womensbrainhealth.org/come-to-think-of-it/7-stages-of-alzheimers-7-levels-of-dementia> [accessed 19 December 2018].

[160] 'Stages of Alzheimer's'.

[161] 'Clinical Stages of Alzheimer's', *Fisher Center for Alzheimer's Research Foundation*, 2014 <https://www.alzinfo.org/understand-alzheimers/clinical-stages-of-alzheimers/> [accessed 19 December 2018].

[162] 'Stages of Dementia', *Queensland Brain Institute*, 2017 <https://qbi.uq.edu.au/dementia/stages-dementia> [accessed 19 December 2018].

[163] 'Late Stage Dementia – What Might You Expect?', *The Unforgettable Blog*, 2015 <https://www.unforgettable.org/blog/late-stage-dementia-what-might-you-expect/> [accessed 19 December 2018].

[164] 'The Later Stages of Dementia', *Alzheimer's Society* <https://www.alzheimers.org.uk/about-dementia/symptoms-and-diagnosis/how-dementia-progresses/later-stages> [accessed 19 December 2018].

[165] 'Seven Stages of Dementia | Symptoms, Progression & Durations' <https://www.dementiacarecentral.com/aboutdementia/facts/stages/> [accessed 19 December 2018].

[166] 'Alzheimer's Stages: How the Disease Progresses', *Mayo Clinic* <https://www.mayoclinic.org/diseases-conditions/alzheimers-disease/in-depth/alzheimers-stages/art-20048448> [accessed 19 December 2018].

[167] '2016-Facts-and-Figures.Pdf' <https://www.alz.org/documents_custom/2016-facts-and-figures.pdf> [accessed 18 February 2018].

[168] Rita Guerreiro and Jose Bras, 'The Age Factor in Alzheimer's Disease', *Genome Medicine*, 7 (2015)

<https://doi.org/10.1186/s13073-015-0232-5>.

[169] 'Alcohol and Tobacco - Alcohol Alert No. 39-1998' <https://pubs.niaaa.nih.gov/publications/aa39.htm> [accessed 7 December 2018].

[170] Christi A. Patten, John E. Martin, and Neville Owen, 'Can Psychiatric and Chemical Dependency Treatment Units Be Smoke Free?', *Journal of Substance Abuse Treatment*, 13.2 (1996), 107–18 <https://doi.org/10.1016/0740-5472(96)00040-2>.

[171] 'CDC - Fact Sheets-Alcohol Use And Health - Alcohol', 2018 <https://www.cdc.gov/alcohol/fact-sheets/alcohol-use.htm> [accessed 7 December 2018].

[172] 'WHO | Alcohol', *WHO* <https://www.who.int/substance_abuse/facts/alcohol/en/> [accessed 7 December 2018].

[173] 'CDC - Frequently Asked Questions - Alcohol', 2017 <https://www.cdc.gov/alcohol/faqs.htm> [accessed 19 February 2018].

[174] 'Alcohol-Related Brain Damage', *Alzheimer's Society* <https://www.alzheimers.org.uk/about-dementia/types-dementia/alcohol-related-brain-damage> [accessed 7 December 2018].

[175] Paul R. Albert, 'Why Is Depression More Prevalent in Women?', *Journal of Psychiatry & Neuroscience□: JPN*, 40.4 (2015), 219–21 <https://doi.org/10.1503/jpn.150205>.

[176] 'Depression in Women: Understanding the Gender Gap', *Mayo Clinic* <https://www.mayoclinic.org/diseases-conditions/depression/in-depth/depression/art-20047725> [accessed 8 December 2018].

[177] Archana Singh-Manoux and others, 'Trajectories of Depressive Symptoms Before Diagnosis of Dementia: A 28-Year Follow-up Study', *JAMA Psychiatry*, 74.7 (2017), 712–

18 <https://doi.org/10.1001/jamapsychiatry.2017.0660>.

[178] Breno S. Diniz and others, 'Late-Life Depression and Risk of Vascular Dementia and Alzheimer's Disease: Systematic Review and Meta-Analysis of Community-Based Cohort Studies', *The British Journal of Psychiatry*, 202.5 (2013), 329–35 <https://doi.org/10.1192/bjp.bp.112.118307>.

[179] 'Alzheimer's or Depression: Could It Be Both?', *Mayo Clinic* <https://www.mayoclinic.org/diseases-conditions/alzheimers-disease/in-depth/alzheimers/art-20048362> [accessed 7 December 2018].

[180] Amy L. Byers and Kristine Yaffe, 'Depression and Risk of Developing Dementia', *Nature Reviews. Neurology*, 7.6 (2011), 323–31 <https://doi.org/10.1038/nrneurol.2011.60>.

[181] Raymond L. Ownby and others, 'Depression and Risk for Alzheimer Disease', *Archives of General Psychiatry*, 63.5 (2006), 530–38 <https://doi.org/10.1001/archpsyc.63.5.530>.

[182] 'Alzheimer's Disease - Symptoms and Causes', *Mayo Clinic* <http://www.mayoclinic.org/diseases-conditions/alzheimers-disease/symptoms-causes/syc-20350447> [accessed 19 February 2018].

[183] 'Alzheimer's Disease & Down Syndrome', *NDSS* <https://www.ndss.org/resources/alzheimers/> [accessed 4 December 2018].

[184] 'Aging-and-Down-Syndrome.Pdf' <http://www.ndss.org/wp-content/uploads/2017/11/Aging-and-Down-Syndrome.pdf> [accessed 4 December 2018].

[185] 'NDSS_Guidebook_FINAL.Pdf' <http://www.ndss.org/wp-content/uploads/2017/11/NDSS_Guidebook_FINAL.pdf> [accessed 9 December 2018].

[186] 'Alzheimer's Disease & Down Syndrome', *NDSS* <https://www.ndss.org/resources/alzheimers/> [accessed 9 December 2018].

[187] 'How Does Alzheimer's Affect Women and Men Differently? | Cognitive Vitality | Alzheimer's Drug Discovery Foundation' <https://www.alzdiscovery.org/cognitive-vitality/blog/how-does-alzheimers-affect-women-and-men-differently> [accessed 7 December 2018].

[188] Martin Prince and others, 'Recent Global Trends in the Prevalence and Incidence of Dementia, and Survival with Dementia', *Alzheimer's Research & Therapy*, 8.1 (2016), 23 <https://doi.org/10.1186/s13195-016-0188-8>.

[189] Jessica L. Podcasy and C. Neill Epperson, 'Considering Sex and Gender in Alzheimer Disease and Other Dementias', *Dialogues in Clinical Neuroscience*, 18.4 (2016), 437–46 <https://www.ncbi.nlm.nih.gov/pmc/articles/PMC5286729/> [accessed 9 December 2018].

[190] 'Scientists Shed New Light on Gender Differences in Alzheimer's', *BrightFocus Foundation*, 2017 <https://www.brightfocus.org/alzheimers/news/scientists-shed-new-light-gender-differences-alzheimers> [accessed 9 December 2018].

[191] 'Assessing Risk for Alzheimer's Disease', *National Institute on Aging* <http://www.nia.nih.gov/health/assessing-risk-alzheimers-disease> [accessed 19 February 2018].

[192] Lars Bertram and Rudolph E. Tanzi, 'Thirty Years of Alzheimer's Disease Genetics: The Implications of Systematic Meta-Analyses', *Nature Reviews Neuroscience*, 9.10 (2008), 768–78 <https://doi.org/10.1038/nrn2494>.

[193] 'Early-Onset Alzheimer's: Symptoms, Diagnosis, and Treatment', *Medical News Today*

<https://www.medicalnewstoday.com/articles/315247.php> [accessed 9 December 2018].

[194] 'Alzheimer's Disease Genetics Fact Sheet', *National Institute on Aging* <https://www.nia.nih.gov/health/alzheimers-disease-genetics-fact-sheet> [accessed 9 December 2018].

[195] Kenny Walter, 'Scientists Identify Genetic Risk Factor for Alzheimer's', *Research & Development*, 2018 <https://www.rdmag.com/article/2018/04/scientists-identify-genetic-risk-factor-alzheimers> [accessed 10 December 2018].

[196] Chengzhong Wang and others, 'Gain of Toxic Apolipoprotein E4 Effects in Human IPSC-Derived Neurons Is Ameliorated by a Small-Molecule Structure Corrector', *Nature Medicine*, 24.5 (2018), 647 <https://doi.org/10.1038/s41591-018-0004-z>.

[197] Emer R. McGrath and others, 'Blood Pressure from Mid- to Late Life and Risk of Incident Dementia', *Neurology*, 89.24 (2017), 2447–54 <https://doi.org/10.1212/WNL.0000000000004741>.

[198] 'AAN' <https://www.aan.com/PressRoom/Home/PressRelease/1660> [accessed 10 December 2018].

[199] 'Hypertension Highlights 2017', 22.

[200] 'More than 100 Million Americans Have High Blood Pressure, AHA Says', *Www.Heart.Org* <https://www.heart.org/en/news/2018/05/01/more-than-100-million-americans-have-high-blood-pressure-aha-says> [accessed 10 December 2018].

[201] 'WHO | Raised Blood Pressure', *WHO* <https://www.who.int/gho/ncd/risk_factors/blood_pressure_prevalence_text/en/> [accessed 10 December 2018].

202 'Risk Factors | Alzheimer Society of Canada' <http://alzheimer.ca/en/Home/About-dementia/Alzheimer-s-disease/Risk-factors> [accessed 19 February 2018].

203 'Frequent Brain Stimulation In Old Age Reduces Risk Of Alzheimer's Disease', *ScienceDaily* <https://www.sciencedaily.com/releases/2007/06/070627161810.htm> [accessed 10 December 2018].

204 Robert S. Wilson and others, 'Participation in Cognitively Stimulating Activities and Risk of Incident Alzheimer Disease', *JAMA*, 287.6 (2002), 742–48 <https://doi.org/10.1001/jama.287.6.742>.

205 Panagiota Mistridis and others, 'Use It or Lose It! Cognitive Activity as a Protec-Tive Factor for Cognitive Decline Associated with Alzheimer's Disease', *Swiss Medical Weekly*, 147.0910 (2017) <https://doi.org/10.4414/smw.2017.14407>.

206 '151-11-1064.Pdf' <https://watermark.silverchair.com/151-11-1064.pdf?token=AQECAHi208BE49Ooan9kkhW_Ercy7Dm3ZL_9Cf3qfKAc485ysgAAAlQwggJQBgkqhkiG9w0BBwaggJBMIICPQIBADCCAjYGCSqGSIb3DQEHATAeBglghkgBZQMEAS4wEQQMDIjEhY8xDH0-DMCPAgEQgIICB3lWtR5-EpPRdmA3Ebh8sgoQeEDNQs8nFCJ0dObkuPlXhq6eQVjEsE37NB6p4IndTkk_XqqVhAy2zDayOp5eMQZF6yAwZyDlVPVszX4tIQPi5_0oPFbW6ODRD0BAdvzPFfuUJzv0aUv9prwmh_0vV4p-1cpp1MGn6smPZSXkq1CkZL9E3Luk4rhQ_tkMjSH4e9yMiP9d2EenyAHW8_Wk4LraH_NXpgP6usnc9cBRAmBQziNcokwnOOyNGpSBCVpVPD70qJZBqdNBS5xdyRhBt30_2T7Prf5cC9UkAZaGXfLvFkzJSz5X4tSFzY3TScQZBScgQTf97PrJ8ZoMmedCMV0fjGmXkAmyvD2nlwlUptOKkEyiOS9LSMPAqcvRNb-EwHJ9ZTczj6l2deeuQetp2721IqB-93FzhE5ZXRhHx9OPQwnpzeyfTuxK3U19-

957bYxZjJTYHiURrk3d4XLr4HB0BptwTN0qKpYquitY0uA LtAprPH9oeI0_v5OyY2Gd39ZG1BbxkY-fy_SQw_y2Fod7CypRFZdBWQdAmnwP-xBPGOuqtM3R2V2vDj6UmU44-9-T8Aqh6Ovd5_OfVqOlVrgkGIZQfahgGHAfCWQQNrf9N8Y1 gUQNB02EZNmYrAjTkRv75ThvMsyk2KwPcPhU_7CRvZkE uissHgBs_3A_vuVYevnkRAX29Q> [accessed 10 December 2018].

[207] 'Low Education Level Linked To Alzheimer's, Study Shows', *ScienceDaily* <https://www.sciencedaily.com/releases/2007/10/071001172855.htm> [accessed 10 December 2018].

[208] Rachel A Whitmer and others, 'Obesity in Middle Age and Future Risk of Dementia: A 27 Year Longitudinal Population Based Study', *BMJ□: British Medical Journal*, 330.7504 (2005), 1360 <https://doi.org/10.1136/bmj.38446.466238.E0>.

[209] Louis A. Profenno, Anton P. Porsteinsson, and Stephen V. Faraone, 'Meta-Analysis of Alzheimer's Disease Risk with Obesity, Diabetes, and Related Disorders', *Biological Psychiatry*, 67.6 (2010), 505–12 <https://doi.org/10.1016/j.biopsych.2009.02.013>.

[210] Rachel A Whitmer and others, 'Obesity in Middle Age and Future Risk of Dementia: A 27 Year Longitudinal Population Based Study', *BMJ□: British Medical Journal*, 330.7504 (2005), 1360 <https://doi.org/10.1136/bmj.38446.466238.E0>.

[211] Miia Kivipelto and others, 'Obesity and Vascular Risk Factors at Midlife and the Risk of Dementia and Alzheimer Disease', *Archives of Neurology*, 62.10 (2005), 1556–60 <https://doi.org/10.1001/archneur.62.10.1556>.

[212] Nikolaos Scarmeas and others, 'Physical Activity, Diet, and Risk of Alzheimer Disease', *JAMA*, 302.6 (2009),

627–37 <https://doi.org/10.1001/jama.2009.1144>.

[213] Yves Rolland, Gabor Abellan van Kan, and Bruno Vellas, 'Physical Activity and Alzheimer's Disease: From Prevention to Therapeutic Perspectives', *Journal of the American Medical Directors Association*, 9.6 (2008), 390–405 <https://doi.org/10.1016/j.jamda.2008.02.007>.

[214] WEI-WEI CHEN, XIA ZHANG, and WEN-JUAN HUANG, 'Role of Physical Exercise in Alzheimer's Disease', *Biomedical Reports*, 4.4 (2016), 403–7 <https://doi.org/10.3892/br.2016.607>.

[215] Virva Hyttinen and others, 'Risk Factors for Initiation of Potentially Inappropriate Medications in Community-Dwelling Older Adults with and without Alzheimer's Disease', *Drugs & Aging*, 34.1 (2017), 67–77 <https://doi.org/10.1007/s40266-016-0415-9>.

[216] Beverly Merz, 'Benzodiazepine Use May Raise Risk of Alzheimer's Disease', *Harvard Health Blog*, 2014 <https://www.health.harvard.edu/blog/benzodiazepine-use-may-raise-risk-alzheimers-disease-201409107397> [accessed 19 February 2018].

[217] Harvard Health Publishing, 'Two Types of Drugs You May Want to Avoid for the Sake of Your Brain', *Harvard Health* <https://www.health.harvard.edu/mind-and-mood/two-types-of-drugs-you-may-want-to-avoid-for-the-sake-of-your-brain> [accessed 11 December 2018].

[218] Kathryn Richardson and others, 'Anticholinergic Drugs and Risk of Dementia: Case-Control Study', *BMJ*, 361 (2018), k1315 <https://doi.org/10.1136/bmj.k1315>.

[219] 'Worst Pills' <https://www.worstpills.org/includes/page.cfm?op_id=459> [accessed 11 December 2018].

[220] 'Mayo Clinic Q and A: Impaired Sleep and Risk of Dementia', *Https://Newsnetwork.Mayoclinic.Org*

<https://newsnetwork.mayoclinic.org/discussion/mayo-clinic-q-and-a-impaired-sleep-and-risk-of-dementia/> [accessed 11 December 2018].

[221] Ram A. Sharma and others, 'Obstructive Sleep Apnea Severity Affects Amyloid Burden in Cognitively Normal Elderly. A Longitudinal Study', *American Journal of Respiratory and Critical Care Medicine*, 197.7 (2017), 933–43 <https://doi.org/10.1164/rccm.201704-0704OC>.

[222] Weihong Pan and Abba J. Kastin, 'Can Sleep Apnea Cause Alzheimer's Disease?', *Neuroscience & Biobehavioral Reviews*, 47 (2014), 656–69 <https://doi.org/10.1016/j.neubiorev.2014.10.019>.

[223] Kristine Yaffe and others, 'Sleep-Disordered Breathing, Hypoxia, and Risk of Mild Cognitive Impairment and Dementia in Older Women', *JAMA*, 306.6 (2011), 613–19 <https://doi.org/10.1001/jama.2011.1115>.

[224] BarneysMusicIsGood, *Bobby McFerrin - Don't Worry Be Happy* <https://www.youtube.com/watch?v=yv-Fk1PwVeU> [accessed 22 February 2018].

[225] Sami Piirainen and others, 'Psychosocial Stress on Neuroinflammation and Cognitive Dysfunctions in Alzheimer's Disease: The Emerging Role for Microglia?', *Neuroscience & Biobehavioral Reviews*, 77 (2017), 148–64 <https://doi.org/10.1016/j.neubiorev.2017.01.046>.

[226] 'Do Beta-Amyloids Cause Alzheimers? | Science 2.0', 2014 <https://www.science20.com/news/do_beta_amyloids_cause_alzheimers> [accessed 11 December 2018].

[227] Matthew A. Stults-Kolehmainen and Rajita Sinha, 'The Effects of Stress on Physical Activity and Exercise', *Sports Medicine (Auckland, N.Z.)*, 44.1 (2014), 81–121 <https://doi.org/10.1007/s40279-013-0090-5>.

[228] Linda Mah, Claudia Szabuniewicz, and Alexandra J.

Fiocco, 'Can Anxiety Damage the Brain?', *Current Opinion in Psychiatry*, 29.1 (2016), 56–63 <https://doi.org/10.1097/YCO.0000000000000223>.

[229] 'AAN'.

[230] Harvard Health Publishing, 'Protect Your Brain from Stress', *Harvard Health* <https://www.health.harvard.edu/mind-and-mood/protect-your-brain-from-stress> [accessed 11 December 2018].

[231] Erin K. Saito and others, 'Smoking History and Alzheimer's Disease Risk in a Community-Based Clinic Population', *Journal of Education and Health Promotion*, 6 (2017) <https://doi.org/10.4103/jehp.jehp_45_15>.

[232] 'WorldAlzheimerReport2014.Pdf' <https://www.alz.co.uk/research/WorldAlzheimerReport2014.pdf> [accessed 7 December 2018].

[233] Jose Luchsinger and others, 'Aggregation of Vascular Risk Factors and Risk of Incident Alzheimer's Disease', *Neurology*, 65.4 (2005), 545–51 <https://doi.org/10.1212/01.wnl.0000172914.08967.dc>.

[234] Timothy C. Durazzo, Niklas Mattsson, and Michael W. Weiner, 'Smoking and Increased Alzheimer's Disease Risk: A Review of Potential Mechanisms', *Alzheimer's & Dementia☐ : The Journal of the Alzheimer's Association*, 10.3 0 (2014), S122–45 <https://doi.org/10.1016/j.jalz.2014.04.009>.

[235] Deborah E. Barnes and Kristine Yaffe, 'The Projected Effect of Risk Factor Reduction on Alzheimer's Disease Prevalence', *The Lancet. Neurology*, 10.9 (2011), 819–28 <https://doi.org/10.1016/S1474-4422(11)70072-2>.

[236] 'WHO_NMH_PND_CIC_TKS_14.1_eng.Pdf' <http://apps.who.int/iris/bitstream/handle/10665/128041/WHO_NMH_PND_CIC_TKS_14.1_eng.pdf?sequence=1> [accessed 11 December 2018].

237 American Diabetes Association 2451 Crystal Drive, Suite 900 Arlington, and Va 22202 1-800-Diabetes, 'Statistics About Diabetes', *American Diabetes Association* <http://www.diabetes.org/diabetes-basics/statistics/> [accessed 8 December 2018].

238 'Diabetes' <https://www.who.int/news-room/fact-sheets/detail/diabetes> [accessed 8 December 2018].

239 'The Top 10 Causes of Death' <https://www.who.int/news-room/fact-sheets/detail/the-top-10-causes-of-death> [accessed 8 December 2018].

240 'Schalter Für Zuckertransport Ins Gehirn Entdeckt' <https://www.tum.de/en/about-tum/news/press-releases/detail/article/33322/> [accessed 6 December 2018].

241 Chin Cheng and others, 'Type 2 Diabetes and Antidiabetic Medications in Relation to Dementia Diagnosis', *The Journals of Gerontology: Series A*, 69.10 (2014), 1299–1305 <https://doi.org/10.1093/gerona/glu073>.

242 Zoe Arvanitakis and others, 'Diabetes Mellitus and Risk of Alzheimer Disease and Decline in Cognitive Function', *Archives of Neurology*, 61.5 (2004), 661–66 <https://doi.org/10.1001/archneur.61.5.661>.

243 Wayne Katon and others, 'Depression Increases Risk of Dementia in Patients with Type 2 Diabetes: The Diabetes & Aging Study', *Archives of General Psychiatry*, 69.4 (2012), 410–17 <https://doi.org/10.1001/archgenpsychiatry.2011.154>.

244 Betsy Simmons Hannibal and Attorney, 'How to Write a Living Will', *Www.Nolo.Com* <https://www.nolo.com/legal-encyclopedia/how-write-living-will.html> [accessed 21 November 2019].

245 'Power of Attorney' <https://www.americanbar.org/groups/real_property_trust_estate/resources/estate_planning/power_of_attorney/> [accessed 22 November 2019].

[246] 'Treatment and Management of Lewy Body Dementia', *National Institute on Aging* <https://www.nia.nih.gov/health/treatment-and-management-lewy-body-dementia> [accessed 24 April 2019].

CPSIA information can be obtained
at www.ICGtesting.com
Printed in the USA
LVHW091529270721
693840LV00014B/59